Understanding Psychosis and Schizophrenia

Understanding Psychosis and Schizophrenia

By

Lieuwe de Haan

Cambridge Scholars Publishing

Understanding Psychosis and Schizophrenia

By Lieuwe de Haan

This book first published 2024

Cambridge Scholars Publishing

Lady Stephenson Library, Newcastle upon Tyne, NE6 2PA, UK

British Library Cataloguing in Publication Data
A catalogue record for this book is available from the British Library

ISBN (10): 1-0364-0335-1
ISBN (13): 978-1-0364-0335-5

CONTENTS

Preface vii

Part 1. Introduction psychosis and schizophrenia

1. Psychosis 2
2. People with schizophrenia 8
3. Brief Western history of psychiatry and schizophrenia 15
4. Criticism of the concept of schizophrenia 21

Part 2. Classification and diagnostics

5. Classification of psychotic disorders 26
6. Diagnosis of vulnerability and resilience 35

Part 3. Scientific research

7. Concepts in scientific research 42
8. Research in psychosis and schizophrenia 56

Part 4. Epidemiology and course

9. Epidemiology of schizophrenia spectrum disorders 62
10. Increased risk 67
11. (Very) early onset Schizophrenia in childhood 71
12. Schizophrenia developing later in life 76
13. (Social) cognitive problems 81

Part 5. Risk factors and underlying mechanisms

14. Genes 92
15. Psychosocial risk factors 105
16. Basic sense of self and psychosis 112
17. Biological risk factors 119
18. Brain 125
19. Dopamine and psychosis 136

20. Glutamate 153
21. Stress 155
22. Neurophysiology 160
23. Immune system 164

Part 6. Other psychiatric or physical problems besides psychosis

24. Anxiety 170
25. Depression 175
26. Trauma 180
27. Addiction 185
28. Obsessions and / or compulsions 194
29. Mental disability 198
30. Autism 200
31. ADHD 204
32. Personality Traits 208
33. Metabolic syndrome 210
34. Movement disorders 214

Part 7. Treatment

35. Personal recovery 222
36. Functional recovery, rehabilitation and stigma 225
37. Family treatment 229
38. Contact with fellow sufferers 232
39. Early intervention in Psychosis 235
40. Psychoeducation 240
41. Antipsychotic medication 242
42. Psychotherapy 272
43. Physical activity 287
44. Neurostimulation 291

PREFACE

If something is bothering you, it is usually good to know a lot about it. Sometimes that can be confronting, but it can also give you grip. In this book I will present current knowledge about psychosis and schizophrenia spectrum disorders. The book is written for patients and their loved ones, who want to learn more about psychosis and schizophrenia. It is also suitable for others, such as teachers, nurses, medical students or doctors. This book gives you an impression of how psychiatrists and researchers think about psychosis and schizophrenia spectrum disorders and what scientific research has yielded so far. Knowledge about occurrence, symptoms, causes, mechanisms and treatment.

It is important for any reader to know from which perspective this book has been written. After all, medicine, psychiatry, science, and authors are not value-free. That is why I write about my point of view in this introduction. Of course there are other valuable points of view, but you will not find them here. This book is written from a medical, scientific and "Western" perspective. In short, I believe that the scientific method is the best we have to understand and improve the world and our relation with the world. The nice thing about the scientific method is that it is critical, stimulates doubt and (if all goes well) prevents ideological positions. Science, as mentioned, is not value-free, and scientists bring their own beliefs and blind spots with them. But they should be critical of themselves and others. I think that knowledge of biology is valuable, but in my opinion many researchers place a lot of emphasis on it. To better understand psychosis, we need science from different perspectives: psychological, biological and social. And we need quantitative and qualitative research. Furthermore, I believe that medicine can often bring limited, yet significant improvements. I think that psychiatric symptoms are scattered in the population and that we make classifications that are more or less correct and that can be meaningful. I also think that our biological and psychological qualities give us possibilities, but also vulnerabilities. We need to take our vulnerabilities into account. Antipsychotics can help in case of psychosis and schizophrenia, however, they have also disadvantages and other help or support is clearly needed. And, maybe most importantly, I think it matters a lot how someone deals with their possibilities and vulnerabilities.

Now you have an idea of where this book comes from.

Schizophrenia and psychosis are complex, and there is still a lot of uncertainty about them. There is also substantial variation in symptoms: they do not manifest themselves in the same way in everyone. Many of the findings are debated. In addition to uncertainty and differences of opinion, there is fortunately also considerable agreement. My goal is to make the available scientific and clinical knowledge accessible to patients, their loved ones and other interested parties. Mind you, much of the information in this book is about backgrounds and causes. If you especially need more practical information, you can find it in Part 1 Chapter 1 and Chapter 2, and in Part 6 and Part 7.

I hope that the knowledge described helps in understanding and overcoming or reducing problems. And that it helps to make decisions about treatment. So that you can use not only your experiential expertise, but also knowledge based on research.

The word patient is used frequently in this book. I talk about patients with schizophrenia or psychosis and about people with schizophrenia or psychosis. A patient is someone who suffers from a medical or psychological problem that creates difficulties in functioning for which professional help is appropriate. Now, of course, someone is not just, or mainly, a patient. But the role of patient suits all of us. It can also refer to any future status. For example, we are all patients of our General Practicioner. By using the word patient, I absolutely do not mean that someone should wait and see what the professional has to offer. On the contrary, the book is actually aimed at strengthening patients and their loved ones with knowledge.

Not surprisingly the term schizophrenia is common in this book. The concept schizophrenia is discussed in more detail in a number of chapters, but I would like to say a few things about it here. Schizophrenia is associated with stigma. This stigma is linked to the prejudice that most people with schizophrenia do not get better and that many of them are dangerous. Both are wrong. The classification of schizophrenia has been wrongly linked to pessimism. It's not a serious brain disease, and it usually doesn't go from bad to worse. It is also problematic that many psychiatrists and scientists themselves also have a pessimistic view of schizophrenia. This may be because some psychiatrists mainly see people with the most severe form of schizophrenia. This gives them the false impression that things usually end badly. Some patients and their loved ones suffer a lot from the classification of schizophrenia and the prejudices that prevail about it. It has made them angry or sad. Moreover, it is clear that it is not easy to distinguish schizophrenia from other psychotic disorders. The causes of schizophrenia are not essentially different from the causes of other psychotic (or even other psychiatric) conditions. For example, we are increasingly aware that variation in genes is associated with various psychiatric disorders. In addition, there is also no specific treatment that is only applicable to people with schizophrenia. In short, critics emphasize that schizophrenia is a concept that carries stigma and they argue that schizophrenia promises specificity, but does not deliver on that promise.

So, critics say: get rid of that word, because schizophrenia does not exist. They are right: schizophrenia does not exist. Just like Parkinson's disease or depression doesn't exist. All patients with Parkinson's disease and all patients with depression are different from each other. The causes can differ, the course differs and the therapy differs. Just like with schizophrenia. Diseases are "constructs," that is, they are human-made. On the basis of agreement between experts these constructs are defined. Psychiatrists have a set criteria for classifying schizophrenia, and if a problem someone has meets those criteria, then that person's psychiatric problem is called schizophrenia. It doesn't exist, we invented it. We agreed on the concept.

However, should we stop using the word "schizophrenia"? Does that solve the problem of stigma? Do we no longer have any difficulty in distinguishing between the different problems of different people? Is "psychotic disorder" a better term? Can we convince the rest of the world to get rid of the word schizophrenia?

I think the answer to all these questions is negative. We don't improve patients' prospects if we rename their problem. People are very different from each other and we have to take this into account in the treatment. Psychosis is common, with other conditions or without causing problems. Placing all psychotic disorders, including schizophrenia under the heading of "psychotic disorder" ignores an important feature of the problems of people who now meet the criteria of schizophrenia. Namely: that they have been suffering from psychotic symptoms for quite some time. And that that indicates a rather persistent and substantial vulnerability.

From previous research, we know that schizophrenia is variable and sometimes difficult to define. Still, it is good that researchers continue to work on schizophrenia. It is an advantage that recently the concept of "schizophrenia spectrum disorders" has been introduced and that more attention is being paid to different symptom dimensions and that we are aware of the problems with the term schizophrenia. But internationally the term schizophrenia is still used and there is still no agreement on a better term.

“Schizophrenia” describes a psychotic disorder that has existed for more than six months and is associated with obvious problems in functioning. The long-term burden is built into the classification. We know that for people who meet the criteria for schizophrenia that the risk of a psychotic relapse is high. And therefore, we know that it is worth taking this into account in the treatment.

In short, schizophrenia is seen as a term that describes vulnerability. Something to keep in mind. Recognizing that for many patients the outlook is quite good, but that a significant proportion of them require continued support and that for the vast majority of patients the vulnerability remains.

Finally, a few less tricky points. “He” and “she” are used interchangeably. Furthermore, I have tried to avoid technical concepts as much as possible. Sometimes I couldn’t avoid it. Then I tried to describe these terms as clearly as possible.

What is this book not about?

It is also important to clarify what the book is not about. It is not about how you cope with feelings, emotions, worries and meaning. It’s not about dealing with loss, or how exactly you build or regain your confidence. These questions are very important, but they are also very personal. I do not consider myself able to write about that in general sense. This book is also not about assistance with housing, education, work, finances or relationships. All very important subjects, but not the focus of this book.

In addition, I would like to emphasize that findings from research often only apply to average patients, while hardly anyone is “average”. Sometimes the text is too rosy. Sometimes the text is too gloomy. The book is not exactly about you. If you are left with questions: discuss them with your friends or professional caregiver.

December 2023, Lieuwe de Haan

PART 1.

INTRODUCTION PSYCHOSIS AND SCHIZOPHRENIA

CHAPTER 1

PSYCHOSIS

What is a psychosis?

Psychosis can be a lot of different things. Psychosis is captivating, special, terrifying, fantastic, terrible, funny, serious, deadly, reassuring, impressive, admirable, sick, incomprehensible, scary, original, annoying, maddening, beautiful, depressiony, handsome, lonely, inspiring, understandable, and moving. Of course, it cannot be all that at the same time. One thing is clear: psychosis varies considerably and the differences between people with psychosis are enormous.

What are the characteristics of a psychosis?

So many people, so many psychoses. Psychosis concerns what we think, how we think and what we perceive. A psychosis is a state in which the belief, thinking or processing of perceptions differs from normal. But that does not immediately make it clearer. Because what is normal? Is it normal to think that young people should always listen to the elderly? Is it normal to think that healthcare does not have to be accessible to everyone? Is it normal to think that you should make as much money as possible? Is it normal to believe in telepathy? Is it normal to think you have to kill unbelievers? Is it normal to believe that horoscopes provide valuable information? Many people do not think so, but many others are fully convinced of it. What is true or normal for one person, is not true or normal for another.

When do we consider a thought, a way of thinking or an observation as normal and when as a psychotic phenomenon? Psychosis has a number of characteristics. None of these features allow an absolute distinction between what is and what is not psychotic. But taken together, these features are used to determine that a thought or perception is psychotic. These characteristics, which I discuss below, are:

1 You stand alone in your thought or perception.
2 Your thought or perception is considered not to be realistic.

3 You remain convinced of your thought or perception, despite evidence to the contrary.
4 You or others are hindered by your thoughts or perceptions.

Incidentally, not only "what" you think can be psychotic, "how" you think can also be psychotic. Criteria for this are:

1 Others do not understand what you mean, they cannot follow you properly.
2 Your way of thinking is illogical or you form new concepts that have never been conceived by anyone else.
3 Your way of thinking remains difficult to follow for a longer period of time.
4 Your way of thinking is disturbing to yourself or to others.

So, one of the characteristics of a psychosis is that there is really only one person who has a certain thought or belief, or perceives something in a certain way. You are alone in your thoughts and/or observations. No one else shares them. No one else can track it. Nobody else believes you. That is very lonely. You are on your own. But this characteristic, standing alone, is not conclusive either. The first to think that the earth was round was also completely on his own. Still, he had no psychotic idea, but, on the contrary, was right. And on the other hand, sometimes a charismatic person has strange or dangerous ideas that are completely adopted by a number of followers. For example, there have been sects whose members killed themselves because they believed, like their leader, that the world would end on a specific date. We then think that that group of people have all adopted a delusion. But this is rare. The vast majority of people with a psychosis are on their own. No one can follow what you experience, no one else shares your beliefs.

Another characteristic of psychosis is that the thought or perception are not real. According to others, the psychotic thought or perception cannot be right. You are not chased by the intelligence service, others cannot read your mind, the neighbor does not talk to you when you hear his voice. But you can sometimes argue about that characteristic too. Because what is reality? How do we know for sure that telepathy doesn't exist? Moreover, people often see how you feel from your face or posture. At least, they think they know your feelings. Then, you could argue, it is only a small step to being able to read someone's thoughts? Sometimes it is clear: if you think half of your brain has been pulverized, then almost everyone thinks that is unrealistic. But often it is less clear: some people talk behind your back, but it is very unlikely that very large groups of people are talking about you.

According to the two characteristics discussed, in a psychosis you have individual thoughts or perceptions that others label as unrealistic. But we all have unrealistic ideas every day, and they are not counted as psychotic ideas. A characteristic of a psychotic idea is that it is an important idea to you and that it is not possible to be dissuaded from it. Others can try, but you remain convinced. In fact, the more others try to convince you that your idea is wrong, the more convinced you become that your idea is really true. As a result, you will increasingly be alone. This characteristic - the unshakable conviction - is also common among people who hold certain beliefs, for instance religious ideas. But often they share it with others. These people usually never change their minds, but as said: someone with a psychotic idea has a strong conviction and is alone in it.

The last characteristic is that you or others are hindered by your beliefs, your way of thinking or your perceptions. For example, you may avoid contact with other people because you think they can read your mind. Or you can destroy your phone because you think it has been hacked. Or you can no longer concentrate on a conversation because you keep hearing voices.

To summarize, a psychotic thought, way of thinking or perception must simultaneously meet four characteristics:

1 You stand alone in your thought or perception.
2 Your thought or perception is not realistic.
3 You hold on to your thought or perception, despite attempts to convince you otherwise.
4 You or others are hindered by your thought or perception.

None of these characteristics in itself allows an absolute distinction. And the assessment is arbitrary. It is work of humans. Psychiatrists sometimes also discuss whether a phenomenon is psychotic or not.

What kind of psychotic symptoms are there?

Psychosis can manifest itself in three different phenomena:

1 It can be the content of your thoughts. So, <u>what</u> you think. Psychotic thoughts are called delusions.

2 It can concern your experiences. You can perceive something while your senses are not receiving stimuli. Such experiences are called hallucinations
3 Finally, it can concern your way of thinking. So, how you think. Your train of thought cannot be followed by others. Your train of thought may suddenly stop. Or you associations are difficult to follow by others.

What are delusions?

Delusions are beliefs that are unrealistic, not shared by those around you, and cannot be dissuaded. There are different types of delusions. Paranoid delusions are common. You have the idea that others are chasing you, are bad for you or are forming a conspiracy. With delusions of grandeur, you are convinced that you are very special, have special gifts or will soon become famous. That is a nice dream, and it does not have to be so much of a nuisance to yourself. In delusions of reference you think that all kinds of things you see or hear have a special meaning for you. You think that messages on television or billboards have a special meaning for yourself. You can also be convinced that someone or something interferes with your thoughts. Or that thoughts are inserted in your head, or withdrawn from your head. Or that your thoughts are broadcasted. Sometimes people think that a chip has been inserted into their head or body that affects them. With somatic delusions you are convinced that something is wrong in your body. For example, that you have sharp objects in your blood vessels or that your brain is swelling. With nihilistic delusions you are convinced that you are worthless or even not exist. In melancholic delusions you think you are guilty of misery and accidents in the world.

What are Hallucinations?

Hallucinations are experiences of a perception without the relevant sense being stimulated. So, you hear a voice (or music or some other sound) while no sound vibrations come to your eardrum. You hear that you are being spoken to, but no one around you is speaking.

Hallucinations can also involve other sensory experiences. You can see images while no light hits your retina. Or smell a scent when there is no volatile substance reaching the nerve cells in the back of your nose. Or you can taste a flavor without your taste buds coming into contact with a particular substance. Or feeling something without being touched.

A hallucination is a real experience of a perception. You really hear, see, smell, taste or feel something. Only the corresponding sense is not stimulated. Your brain is kidding you. They register an observation and that is why you experience it. That experience feels real.

What is confused thinking?

Confused thinking or disorganization means that your thinking is no longer logical. At least not easy to follow for someone else. These problems are also referred to as "formal thinking disorders". Of course, psychiatrists cannot really judge your thinking. They only can listen to what you say, and on that basis, they judge how you think. You may be jumping from one subject to another, it is not clear how or why you switch from one topic to another. Or your thinking may seem chaotic or go too fast or too slow. Sometimes your train of thought can suddenly be interrupted. The formation of new words is also counted as a formal thought disorder. Sometimes people with schizophrenia come up with very powerful, striking new words. One patient told a colleague, whom he was apparently not very satisfied with, that he was not a psychiatrist, but a "psych hater". In this case you could also say that someone is very creative with language. In addition, the disorganization can also manifest itself in confused behavior.

With what can you compare psychosis?

A psychosis is a state in which the processing of information is disturbed and which leads to psychotic symptoms: delusions, hallucinations and/or confusion. You could compare psychosis with fever. Fever is a phenomenon that can occur with various illnesses. Fever indicates increased activity in your body. Psychosis can also occur in various psychiatric conditions and indicates increased mental activity and disturbed processing of information. People with depression can become psychotic, just like people who use cocaine. And if you have had surgery and are still drowsy from the anesthesia, and if your hearing aid is off and you miss your glasses, you can also get psychosis. When the psychotic state has a physical cause and your consciousness is disturbed, we speak of a delirium.

However, you can also have psychotic symptoms without causing problems. For example, some people occasionally hear voices when no one is speaking to them. But they don't suffer from that; they don't find it disturbing. In fact, they often take what is being said as a good advice. Then these psychotic symptoms do not occur in the context of a disorder. So, you can have psychotic symptoms without having a psychiatric condition.

What is the difference between psychosis and schizophrenia?

There may be confusion about the distinction between psychosis and schizophrenia.

Psychosis, as explained, is a state in which the processing of information is disturbed and which leads to psychotic symptoms: delusions, hallucinations and / or confusion. Schizophrenia is a classification in which someone suffers from a psychosis impacting on social functioning, with a number of other characteristics and a duration of the problems of at least six months.

The comparison is not entirely correct, but you could say that psychosis is "fever" and schizophrenia is "pneumonia". Psychosis is a phenomenon and a symptom. Schizophrenia is an indication of a certain "vulnerability or condition".

What is meant by Positive Symptoms?

This is a somewhat strange term. You may initially think of something beneficial. But it simply means that there are symptoms that are not normally present in someone. It is something new, something extra on top of the normal state. Consider, for example, delusions, hallucinations or symptoms of disorganization: normally someone does not have these kinds of problems, but they do now. If one or more of these symptoms are present to a sufficiently severe degree, we speak of positive symptoms.

What is meant by Negative Symptoms?

Unlike positive symptoms, negative symptoms do not indicate excess, but rather a deficiency, something that is missing. Something that is normally there, is now less present or absent altogether. Normally you see emotions on people's faces. Normally people use gestures. Normally people move. Normally people are motivated. Normally people worry. There are negative symptoms when these kinds of normal things are no longer present. For example, people with negative symptoms show less initiative, barely speak, have difficulty taking action and show little emotions. They are often bored and feel a void. Their urge to do something is limited, they hardly have spontaneous thoughts or they experience a decrease in creativity. Lying in bed for a long time, looking straight ahead without thinking, not going to school or work, paying little attention to grooming are all examples of the consequences of negative symptoms.

CHAPTER 2

PEOPLE WITH SCHIZOPHRENIA

This chapter is about how people with schizophrenia view schizophrenia. To this end, I have compiled an anthology of impressive stories I encountered. I changed names and circumstances, to avoid recognition. These stories show how different people think about the difficulties and the possibilities, and they give an impression of important themes in their life. Finally, I will mention some famous people with schizophrenia.

What is schizophrenia according to people who have experience with it?

Paul: "The stigma on schizophrenia is huge. You can overcome that by being open. But schizophrenia is also one of the most cruel illnesses out there. I got depressed and had bad voices a lot. I was also extremely anxious, and I didn't even dare to leave the house because of the voices. I heard several, both from acquaintances and strangers. They said, "We're going to do bad things to you." Sometimes the voices make me seem absent, because I have to have two discussions at the same time. One in my head and one with an outsider. I have learned to handle voices better and I don't pay a lot attention to it anymore. It is a short circuit in the brain, no more, no less. Nowadays the voices are more in the background and are more positive. I am stronger than the voices!

In my opinion, doctors have a duty to engage in psychoeducation and recovery. Prescribing pills alone is absolutely not the solution: you have to look for the right treatment together with the patient.

Fortunately, I am doing very well. This is largely due to my mentality and the fact that I have developed myself as a person. I also have a close circle of friends and have received a lot of support from my family. Recently I was hired as a sponsor recruiter at a tennis club. My job is to maintain existing relationships, recruit new sponsors and receive sponsors at the club. So, a lot of social contact, and that goes well for me. "

Jennifer: "The alarm clock rings at 7:30 in the morning" or actually four different alarm clocks go off. And yet that doesn't mean I'm waking up, no matter how badly I want to. Because of the medication I sleep very deeply.

At the station I am always a bit anxious about whether the trains will run that day. The tones that always sound just before an announcement follows, already makes me nervous. I quickly get upset when things don't go according to a set pattern. The filter in my head that separates important impulses from unimportant impulses doesn't work as well as it does in other people. I quickly get tired of many impressions.

I work one half day a week as a board member of a patient association. We used to say we were the nationwide patient association for people with schizophrenia. Today we call it psychosis sensitivity. Our members feel more comfortable with this new name. All the people who work for the patient association have a psychotic disorder themselves. As a result, we understand each other very well. When I tell other people that I work for such an association, I sometimes experience that people think that I am a kind of social worker who supports the organization. People often cannot imagine that our association is run by fellow sufferers, and that for about twenty years! People with schizophrenia can do more than most people think.

Sometimes I am also asked to lecture on schizophrenia. I like to do things like this, because I notice that a lot is still unknown about schizophrenia and that a lot of nonsense is also written and told in the media. I have made it a kind of mission for myself to contribute to a better image of schizophrenia. That also gives direction to my life; I have the feeling that I contribute something. That is why I have also written a book for young people who in one way or another come into contact with schizophrenia.

It remains amazing how a few pills can make a whole psychosis disappear! And moreover, since I started talking about childhood trauma with my psychologist, I have less burden of the symptoms of schizophrenia. But of course, that could also be due to the fact that I am approaching forty: it seems that symptoms are getting milder then. "

Thomas: "I quit my history studies. I was no longer able to attend lectures, because people could read my mind. Just think how awful that is. I completely lost my privacy. Everything you think is on the street. If you think "He has a lot of pimples" or "That's an attractive girl" or "I do want to have sex", it is immediately public. I therefore tried to control my thoughts. Not to think what could be offensive. But that got me completely stuck. I went to the psychiatrist and was persuaded to take antipsychotics. My fear that people could read my mind diminished. I resumed my studies, went back to playing basketball and felt good. At one point my psychiatrist spoke to me about my psychotic period. But we didn't understand each other when he talked about "reading thoughts as a phenomenon of psychosis." There was confusion with both of us. Then I suddenly got it "Oh now I get what you mean: people can only read my mind when I'm psychotic. The belief I had about reading minds is so impressive that it must have been true. I see psychosis as a vulnerability in which my thoughts can be read. "

Jessica: "I see messages related to me everywhere. Those messages tell me how I am doing. It's always right. I see it in advertising and hear it from people on the street, and what I see or hear fits exactly with how I feel. It annoys me, it keeps racing in my head. I've been taking antipsychotics for a long time. It does muffle a bit, but I keep seeing all those things. It is not always bothersome or unpleasant, I also learn things about myself from the things I see. But it is not good for my self-confidence. I think I have schizophrenia. It is a handicap. It makes me feel lonely. "

Barbara: "My parents are very bad for me. They use a lot of drugs and alcohol. My mother especially yells at me. I don't trust anyone anymore. I don't want to go back home, but I don't want to be admitted either. In the evening I hear voices. Usually, they say shitty things. I turn up the music. That helps. A little. The social workers are in league with my parents. Then I have to take pills, while the problem lies with my parents. I don't have schizophrenia. They just say that to hold on to me and make money off me."

Patrick: "Health is a sliding scale. Hearing voices is just as exhausting as a child pulling your sleeve 24 hours a day and asking, "Why?" Or, "When are we going there?" Or: "Are we there yet?" In the early years the voices came from outside forces and often left me defeated. How did they know and why had I not thought of it before? My psychiatrist certainly helped me by making things clearer to me. But in the end, I am the one who knows myself best. I could see the voices more and more as my own. Now the voices advise me: they urge me to run, sometimes stubbornly, but now I believe it is me. I sometimes wonder: What if I got even healthier, would I miss the voices?

Michael: "I am afraid that I will spread a terrible odor. I only dare to go outside with a lot of deodorant. When I hear people talking on the street, I always think they are talking about me. When I concentrate heavily on my work, it fades into the background. But that does not always work.

Sometimes I spend hours listening to what people say on the street. I don't want pills. The doctor says I have a psychosis. Maybe so. I also quit smoking. I no longer use drugs at festivals either. I want to keep thinking clearly."

Emily: "I think I have schizophrenia and it is a brain disorder. But that is not the whole, and certainly not the most important, story. Because the psychotic symptoms have meaning and they have helped me to organize my new life. I have seen that some patients can really get better from antipsychotics, but others get worse nevertheless. Antipsychotics only treat part of the problem. I heard many voices. I was chaotic, often depressed. I was on antidepressants, but I remained depressed. One day I heard voices from birds saying, "We love you Emily." Later I heard a clear voice: "Believe in Jesus and everything will be all right." Since then, I had a direction in my life and people started helping me. And I became less chaotic. I think God can speak to you through psychosis. Atheist psychiatrists don't believe that, but they are wrong. My psychosis made me know which way to go. "

Sarah: "After my divorce, I started to notice that the neighbors looked in a special way when I walked by. Often, they turned around quickly. I also heard them laugh behind my back. When I wanted to go to sleep, they started making noises on purpose. I think they also entered my house. Then they moved things in my house. I couldn't find anything anymore. My doctor says I am confused. It may be, but I think you better be on your guard. He consulted a psychiatrist, and now I am on antipsychotics before sleeping. I sleep better. Whether I have a psychosis? I do not know. In any case, I want to keep living on my own. "

Susan: "Making friends is as difficult as landing a capsule on Jupiter. I know all the ingredients. But maybe I'm too shy, they think I'm boring, I can't keep the conversation going… When I'm on medication I'm stable and balanced. I benefit a lot from my family. They accept me as I am. And I also have some friends that I see a few times a year. But I don't really have someone I see every week or just call me to go out. And if that doesn't work, how am I supposed to find a partner? Do I want children? Of course, I want children. But I'm also afraid they could get schizophrenia. Can I raise them without damaging them? I am happy with everything I have, although I am often afraid of losing it. I wish I had more, enough to land a capsule on Jupiter."

Nancy: "My son jumped off a building just before his 34th birthday. I miss him so much. He grew in me and I have always cherished him. He liked to surf. We lost him since he was 21. He withdrew. Threw away the food I brought because he was afraid of being poisoned. He took his medication. He wanted to get better. But nothing helped. It also made him desperate. He shouted, "I'm not taking my medication because I'm sick, I'm sick because I'm taking medication!"

Musaf: "I have schizophrenia. If I don't take clozapine, my thoughts get restless, I start paying more and more attention to all the insidious things that happen. This is going from bad to worse. I then pace, feel furious and helpless. I used to be separated. I have had severe psychosis three times. I never want to experience that again. That's why I take clozapine. It bothers me nevertheless. I sleep around the clock and it takes quite a long time in the morning before I feel a little clear. Do agree with my psychiatrist. I am really sensitive to psychosis."

Linda: "I want to emphasize the importance of psychotherapy. My previous professional caregiver gave me too much antipsychotics, and he was judgmental. Now I use a lot less drugs, and my psychiatrist is calm, open and friendly. My psychoses have a lot to do with trauma that I have suffered. Also, psychological trauma. Precisely everything I've been through has made me more suspicious. It helps me a lot to be able to talk about this. That I'm being listened to. I don't dare to do that with people I know. It took a lot of time. You cannot quickly recover from broken trust. But through psychotherapy I work on myself. My psychiatrist doesn't have to do much, just ask the right questions, support me, and be patient. Then I get better. "

Daniel: "I am now 44 years old and fully recovered from schizophrenia. From the age of 20 I have been admitted to a psychiatric hospital ten times. I have not used antipsychotics since I was 37. I thought my thoughts could influence things in the world. My train of thought was difficult for an ordinary mortal soul to follow. I was very sensitive to everything that was going on around me. I dropped out of college and they told me I would never recover. But that's nonsense: I've recovered. You can be cured of schizophrenia. I became an artist and I still have special gifts.

Changing my lifestyle brought about my recovery. I have slowly tapered off the drugs and am on a vegetarian diet. A lot of fat helps me: I usually eat 250 grams of French cheese and two avocados a day. I should avoid proteins. I also run a lot, and I always visit friends by bike. And it was important that my friends and family supported me. I am a living proof that you can recover from schizophrenia. "

Aaron: "Belief in Atheism. That's what I've learned. I used to make the choice for life. I did this by not opting for a university study: then I would have become psychotic and suicidal again. So, I chose life and became a social worker. And my belief is that I can mean something to other people and to the world. That belief is my life. I sometimes think that others speak ill of me or that items in the news relate to me. But through yoga and through my faith I get over it. Life without faith is worse than death. "

Which famous people met the schizophrenia classification?

Vaslav Nijinsky (1889-1950) was a famous ballet dancer who was asked to perform all over the world. People were moved to tears by his dance. He married and had two daughters. At the age of 28, he became confused and had fits of rage. He was diagnosed with schizophrenia by Eugen Bleuler and was repeatedly admitted to psychiatric hospitals. In later life he became more balanced.

Eduard Einstein (1910-1965) was the son of Albert Einstein. He was very smart and musical. He started studying medicine because he wanted to become a psychiatrist. At the age of 20 he was admitted with the symptoms of schizophrenia. He continued to write letters to his father, but Albert Einstein (who emigrated to the United States) never saw his son again. Eduard remained interested in poetry and could play the piano beautifully, but his memory and ability to remember was severely damaged by the many electroshocks he received, according to his brother.

John Forbes Nash (1928-2015) was a genius mathematician. He is the only person to have won both the Nobel Prize in Economics and the Abel Prize (a kind of Nobel Prize in Mathematics). Nash received many honorary degrees and spoke at many congresses.

From the age of 32, he became suspicious and has been repeatedly hospitalized. Nash said his "mental disorders" started when his wife was pregnant. The scientific rationality of his thinking changed to the idea that he saw a messenger or had a special function himself. He felt haunted. A few years later he started to hear voices. He only took antipsychotics when forced to. From the age of 52 his condition improved and he gradually returned to academic work. He later said, "I would not have had good scientific ideas if I had thought more normal." Nash saw schizophrenia as an unacceptable way of thinking. He emphasized the evolutionary benefits of human diversity and apparently absurd behavior.

Nash and his wife had a son. Nash lived with his wife in between psychiatric admissions, even after their divorce. They later remarried. Nash and his wife were killed in 2015 when the taxi they were in crashed.

Syd Barrett (1946-2006) was the founder of Pink Floyd. His father was a famous pathologist. Syd was the singer and main author of the songs that the band released in the early years of its existence. With the first success came the first problems. Barrett's behavior became unpredictable, probably because he used a lot of LSD. David Gilmour, a childhood friend of Syd's, joined the band. It was hoped he could get Syd back on track. In vain: Syd started to use more drugs, got a burnout, heard voices and withdrew from publicity. The last time the members of Pink Floyd saw Syd was when he entered the studio while recording the song "Shine on you crazy diamond," a song about Syd. Coincidence does exist, you would say. Eventually, Syd went back to live with his mother.

Peter Green (1946-2020) is the founder of Fleetwood Mac. He wrote many songs that were also performed by others (Santana, Aerosmith, Status Quo), such as "Albatross" and "Black Magic Woman". Later he suffered from psychosis and was admitted several times, and in the 1970s he received electroconvulsive therapy. After this he regained his balance.

Donny Hathaway (1945-1979) was an American soul singer who could sing beautifully. When he was only four years old, he already performed as a gospelsinger. Hathaway was seen by his colleagues as one of the very best, on par with Aretha Franklin and Ray Charles. He has sung beautiful duets with Roberta Flack, such as "Where is the love" and "The closer I get to you". He also suffered from schizophrenia. During his psychoses he was afraid of being killed by white people and thought his brain was connected to a device that controlled him. At that time, he was smoking a lot and used cocaine. This sometimes made him violent. The relationship with his wife broke down, and after a failed recording day, a day when he also suffered from delusions, he committed suicide at the age of 33. His daughter Lalah Hathaway also later became a famous singer.

References

De Ruijter, Bart and Van Alphen Carola. 2018. "Leven met psychosen en schizofrenie" In Handboek schizofreniespectrumstoornissen, edited by Wiepke Cahn, Inez Myin-Germeys, Richard Bruggeman, Lieuwe de Haan. Amsterdam: De Tijdstroom

CHAPTER 3

BRIEF WESTERN HISTORY OF PSYCHIATRY AND SCHIZOPHRENIA

This chapter focuses on the history of schizophrenia in Western medicine and science. I will not discuss non-Western ideas or cultures. This is certainly not to say that views from other times and cultures cannot be fascinating or helpful. "Madness" is timeless and an impressive phenomenon about which many views and stories exist and existed. Some visions attach importance to prophets, seers, witches, punishment from gods, enchantment and forces of nature. For many people such ideas are meaningful. They can also be supportive for patients and their loved ones, because they do not assume a disease or a disability, but rather something extra that the patient has, something special. That can be a comfort or a confirmation of how they experience it themselves.

How did people feel about psychiatric disorders from ancient times to the eighteenth century?

In ancient times, four natural elements — air, earth, fire, and water — were thought to correspond to bodily fluids: blood, black bile, yellow bile, and mucus. Illness was seen as a disruption of the balance between those fluids. An excess of black bile caused depression or melancholy (literally: black bile). In addition, "phrenitis" was distinguished, in which patients had incorrect sensory perceptions (van den Bosch 2018). Mania was diagnosed when someone was excited and at the same time had a lack of judgment. Until the eighteenth century, three psychiatric disorders were distinguished. They were respectively called melancholy, feverish light-headedness, and madness. The similarity between the different psychiatric conditions was that patients destroyed things that were dear to them or threatened dear people (Haslam 1809).

How did scientific psychiatry start?

As the influence of religion on thinking began to wane, scientists began to describe delusions and hallucinations as symptoms of disease. This was not possible before, because it was believed that experiences and thoughts originated in a supernatural world whose existence was not in question. Gradually there was interest in the inner world and psychology. Some understanding of the functioning of nerve cells was gained and physicians began to accurately describe pathologies and their course. A less strict distinction was also made between "insane" and "normal". Patients could be gripped by a strange passion, but also have moments or periods when they thought normal. Psychiatric illness was thought to arise because the nervous system was unable to maintain proper balance (van den Bosch 2018).

How did scientists and professional caregiver feel about psychological and physical causes in the early eighteenth century?

There was a clear split at the time. Some of the professional caregiver/scientists belonged to so-called romantic speculative psychiatry. They saw no role for physical factors and attached great importance to classifying patients' views. Another part of the professionals was convinced that physical factors were the cause of psychiatric syndromes. Eventually the latter group became more dominant: psychological illnesses came to be viewed in the same way as physical illness and speculative ideas faded into the background. These professionals provided us with careful descriptions of the symptoms and course, and thought that causes of psychiatric disorders could be found in physiology and anatomy (van den Bosch 2018).

How did people think about psychotic disorders at the end of the eighteenth century?

In the late eighteenth century, it was thought that there was one underlying psychotic disorder that could manifest itself in different ways. They tried in vain to classify them on the basis of brain anatomy. It was the German psychiatrist Emil Kraepelin (1856-1926) (see figure 3.1) who suggested distinguishing syndromes on the basis of their course. Kraepelin was strongly influenced by the now outdated idea that there are psychiatric disorders characterized by increasing degeneration (the so-called "degeneration theory"). Kraepelin distinguished dementia praecox from manic-depressive psychoses (Kraepelin 1899).

Figure 3.1 Emil Kraepelin

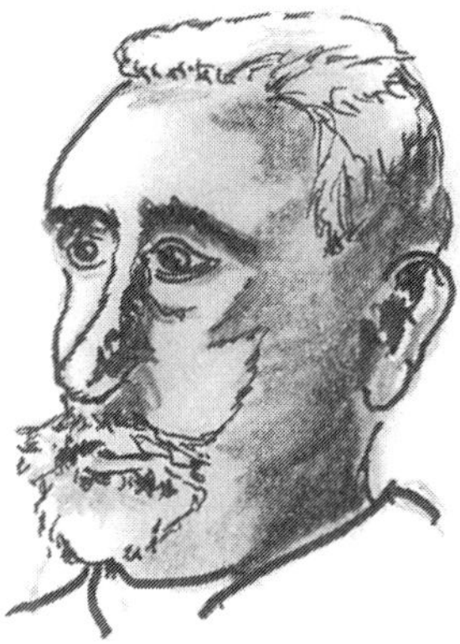

Who introduced the concept of schizophrenia and what did it mean?

Eugen Bleuler (1857-1939) (see figure 3.2) introduced the term schizophrenia and by that he meant the splitting up of psychic functions. He thought the core problem was that correct associations get disturbed, derailing the train of thought. The associations become too much at the mercy of emotions, which makes thoughts too much of the center of attention, reducing the integration of different thoughts (Bleuler 1908, 1911). Daily reality also has less influence on ideas. Bleuler hypothesized that a number of basic symptoms, which all happen to start with an A, are always present in schizophrenia: association disorder, affect disorder, ambivalence, autism, attention and will disorder. He considered delusions, hallucinations and catatonic phenomena as additional symptoms, which therefore do not occur in all patients or always.

Bleuler emphasized that there was a wide variation in severity. That is why an attempt was made to make a categorization within schizophrenia (Bleuler 1908,1911). Kraepelin distinguished, for example, hebephrenia (with many negative symptoms and an unfavorable course), catatonia (with deviations in posture or speech) and paranoia (with delusions and hallucinations). Later he realized that this strict division did not last and he focused more on distinguishing psychic reaction patterns (Kraepelin 1899).

Figure 3.2 Eugen Bleuler

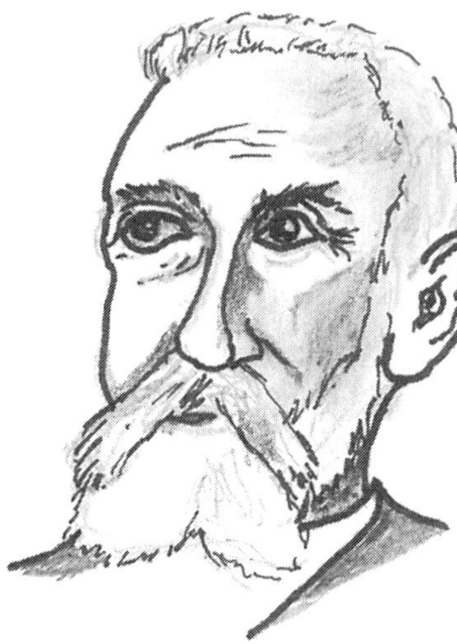

How did the concept of schizophrenia develop in the first half of the twentieth century?

Psychiatrists looked for characteristic symptoms that separate schizophrenia from other psychiatric conditions. They thought of a "thought disorder" or "will disorder", or "a certain sense of alienation that a patient evokes in the researcher". Despite this, the broad label of schizophrenia became applicable to more and more people. Meanwhile, some psychoanalysts developed theories about the cause of the symptoms and the development of schizophrenia, including very erroneous and harmful theories, such as the idea of the sickening role of the mother or the family (van den Bosch 2018).

How did the concept of schizophrenia develop in the second half of the twentieth century?

The Diagnostic and Statistical Manual of Mental Disorders (DSM) was developed in the United States in an effort to achieve greater consensus on different classifications. However, the 1968 DSM-II contained a very broad definition of schizophrenia: Conceptual changes that can lead to misinterpretations of reality and sometimes to delusions and hallucinations (American Psychiatric Association 1968). It was then found that in the United States, many more people are diagnosed with schizophrenia than in

Europe, and stricter diagnostic criteria were proposed. Delusions or hallucinations were characteristic, but not enough.

Psychiatrist Kurt Schneider (1887-1967) (see Figure 3.3) emphasized the importance of the patient's subjective experiences and described what he considered to be the so-called first-order symptoms, i.e. symptoms of which he thought that they were characteristic of schizophrenia: hearing thoughts out loud; voices that speak to or about the patient; thoughts that are entered or removed (Schneider 1959). These ideas influenced the DSM-III-R (the revised version of the third edition of the Diagnostic Handbook), which came out in 1987 (American Psychiatric Association 1987). Another change in the DSM-II-R was that, in contrast to the DSM-II, it was stated that the course of schizophrenia had to be chronic.

Figure 3.3 Kurt Schneider

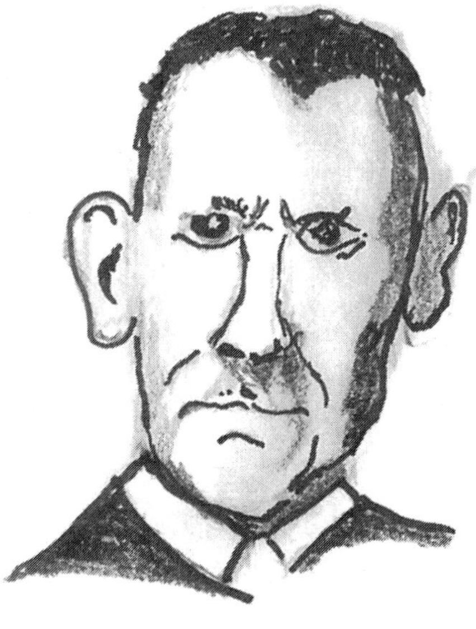

What are the ideas about schizophrenia in the early 21st century?

In general, professional caregiver and scientists are now aware that schizophrenia is a diverse collection of more or less circumscribed conditions, and that there are no characteristic symptoms that occur only in schizophrenia. We now know that it is sometimes difficult to distinguish schizophrenia from other conditions and from normal functioning. The criticism of the concept of schizophrenia is discussed in the next chapter.

The DSM-5 speaks of a spectrum of disorders and attention is paid to different dimensions of symptoms that may be present in schizophrenia spectrum disorders: hallucinations; delusions; disorganization; abnormal psychomotor skills; negative symptoms; cognitive impairments; depression; and mania (American Psychiatric Association 2013).

References

American Psychiatric Association. 1968. Diagnostic and statistical manual of mental disorders (2nd ed.). Washington, DC: American Psychiatric Press.

American Psychiatric Association. 1987. Diagnostic and statistical manual of mental disorders (3rd rev. ed.). Washington, DC: American Psychiatric Press.

American Psychiatric Association. 2013. Diagnostic and statistical manual of mental disorders (5th ed.). Washington: American Psychiatric Press. American Psychiatric Association.

Bleuler, E. 1908. Die Prognose der Dementia praecox (Schizophreniegruppe). Allgemeine Zeitschrift für Psychiatrie und psychischgerichtliche Medizin, 65, 436-464.

Bleuler, E. 1911. Dementia praecox oder Gruppe der Schizophrenien. In G. Aschaffenburg Bosch, R.J. van den. 2018. Gedaanten van de waanzin. Amsterdam: Atheneum.

Haslam, J. 1809. Observations on madness and melancholy (2nd ed.). London: Hayden.

Kraepelin, E. 1899. Zur Diagnose und Prognose der Dementia Praecox. Allgemeine Zeitschrift der Psychiatrie, 56, 254-263.

Schneider, K. 1959. Klinische Psychopathologie (5e Aufl.). Stuttgart: Thieme.

Van den Bosch, Rob. 2018. "Het concept schizofrenie" In Handboek schizofreniespectrumstoornissen, edited by Wiepke Cahn, Inez Myin-Germeys, Richard Bruggeman, Lieuwe de Haan. Amsterdam: De Tijdstroom

CHAPTER 4

CRITICISM OF THE CONCEPT OF SCHIZOPHRENIA

What is the problem with the concept schizophrenia?

The question is whether schizophrenia exists as a specific condition or disease. A disease exists if it is a clearly distinguishable category concerning causes, treatment or prognosis. It is clear that there are major problems with the concept of schizophrenia in these area's (Boyle 2002; Ralston and Blom 2018).

But despite the fact that schizophrenia may not exist in nature, people can use the term as if it does. They see it as something someone has. Or worse, as something someone is. And often also as something that will never pass away or is associated with danger and misery. Schizophrenia is stigmatized. Therefore, there is rightly discussion about the concept (Ralston and Blom 2018).

Why is stigma so nasty?

Some people think that people with schizophrenia are less qualified to take responsibility and that they should not have personal relationships. People with schizophrenia can experience discrimination in the areas of work, education, housing and care. They can also stigmatize themselves and become hopeless and lonely as a result. The view that schizophrenia is a brain disorder, for example, can lead to pessimism: you can then think that it cannot be changed. That is bad for your self-image and self-confidence. Having brain problems does not mean that they are persistent. Everything in our life affects our brains: brains are changeable and can grow and recover. But nonetheless, such persistent associations can add to stigma.

The media often add to the stigma, often linking confused dangerous behavior to psychosis and schizophrenia. Because they hardly ever report on the vast majority of people with psychosis who live their lives calmly and inconspicuously, perhaps somewhat withdrawn and never cause any problems, a distorted image emerges among the general public. However, the idea that schizophrenia is a brain disorder in which your brain reacts too strongly and for too long to stress also has an advantage: it can prevent you from blaming yourself for your problems.

What is the value of the concept of schizophrenia?

The concept of schizophrenia can help professionals and patients to understand and link certain phenomena. It also helps to gain scientific knowledge about causes, treatment and guidance, to bundle matters when problems are somewhat comparable and to be able to discuss them with each other. But there is also a problem here. Are we talking about the same thing? Can we apply knowledge gained from a group of patients to a unique person? By the way, you can ask the same questions for all other psychiatric or medical conditions.

On the basis of the current criteria of schizophrenia, it is a disorder with psychotic symptoms that have a clear impact on functioning, which causes a person to experience discomfort for at least six months.

The value of this category is that it indicates that a person's sensitivity is so substantial that annoying psychotic symptoms have a clear impact and do not disappear quickly. No more and no less. This distinguishes a group of people who suffer from psychotic symptoms for quite a long time. We know of this group that about 80 percent later show psychotic symptoms again. So, it is a group of people in which you have to take into account a high psychosis sensitivity in the longer term. The value of the concept of schizophrenia lies in this observation of a long-lasting sensitivity or vulnerability.

Do you solve the problem of stigma by dropping the concept of schizophrenia?

Scrapping the concept of schizophrenia is not the way to combat the existing stigma in my opinion. Discrimination, generalization, hopelessness, fear and ostracism are unfortunately very common in response to people perceived as "different". If a new name comes along, it will also be stigmatized as soon as problems associated with it arise. In Japan, the old name of schizophrenia, "split mind disease", has been replaced by a new one, the "integration disorder", but unfortunately without clearly diminishing the stigma (Sommer, I., & Carpenter, W.T. 2016).

Are there specific biological abnormalities in schizophrenia?

Extensive research has been done into causes, risk factors and biological abnormalities in schizophrenia. The conclusion is that there are no causes, risk factors or biological abnormalities that only occur in people who meet the schizophrenia criteria (Heinrichs 2001). The value of the concept of schizophrenia therefore does not lie in its biological uniqueness (Ralston and Blom 2018). Fifty years of intensive biological research in psychiatry has not identified any biological abnormality that can be used as a test for any particular psychiatric classification. That is not to say that further biological research into risk factors or underlying mechanisms is meaningless (Sommer and Carpenter 2016). It can certainly help to find answers that apply, to a greater or lesser extent, to people with schizophrenia. It also cannot be ruled out that in the future we will find specific biological causes in some people with schizophrenia. For example, an increased immune response. Then there may be a special effective treatment for that group. So, it is wise to keep looking for causes, even if they only apply to a minority of people with schizophrenia. In any case, it is established that people and their mental functioning are multiform and complex.

References

Boyle, M. 2002. Schizophrenia: A Scientific Delusion? (2nd ed.). London: Routledge.

Heinrichs, R.W. 2001. In search of madness: schizophrenia and neuroscience. Oxford:

Ralston, Alan and Blom, Jan Dirk. 2018. "Kritiek op het schizofrenieconcept" In Handboek schizofreniespectrumstoornissen, edited by Wiepke Cahn, Inez Myin-Germeys, Richard Bruggeman, Lieuwe de Haan. Amsterdam: De Tijdstroom.

Sommer, I., & Carpenter, W.T. 2016. Schizophrenia: changing the name and broadening the concept is problematic. BMJ,352, 1080.

PART 2.

CLASSIFICATION AND DIAGNOSIS

CHAPTER 5

CLASSIFICATION OF PSYCHOTIC DISORDERS

What is Classification?

Classification is the division of phenomena into certain classes or groups on the basis of similarity or relationship in characteristics. Classification is impersonal by definition. You can classify boys and girls, people with black hair or brown or blond hair, or types of soccer players (left legged, right legged, defender, attacker). A classification is by no means the same as a diagnosis.

What is a diagnosis?

Unlike a classification, a diagnosis is personal. A diagnosis describes which complaints someone has and how much influence these complaints have on his/her functioning: which vulnerability was already present, which factors triggered the complaints, which factors contribute to persistence of symptoms. Moreover, in a diagnosis you describe whether someone has specific personality traits, physical factors or whether there is another disease present. And in a diagnosis, you consider stressful circumstances or certain trauma. It is also valuable to include protective factors and strengths in a diagnostic description. The diagnostis describes the relationship between all these factors in one person.

What is the "Diagnostic and Statistical Manual of Mental Disorders" (DSM)?

The Diagnostic and Statistical Manual of Mental Disorders (DSM) is a book that describes characteristics that a problem must have in order to meet the criteria for a particular psychiatric classification (American Psychiatric Association. 1952, 1968, 1982, 1987, 1994, 2013).

What is the purpose of the DSM?

The aim is to establish agreements about the criteria for certain classifications. This increases the chance that two different psychiatrists give the same patient the same classification. This is necessary because previously, psychiatrists used different definitions and different terms for similar psychiatric conditions, which allowed them to arrive at different classifications. The unity of language in psychiatry is largely due to systems such as the DSM (American Psychiatric Association. 1952, 1968, 1982, 1987, 1994, 2013).

What criticism is there of the DSM classification system?

There are many limitations to the DSM and many criticisms. Major limitations include:

1 Many different risk factors apply to several classifications.
2 Symptoms and their course still differ enormously within a specific classification.
3 The course of symptoms and functioning can not be predicted on the basis of a classification.
4 Individual problems and a person's strengths are not addressed in a classification. That is why it is not possible to draw up an individualized care plan based on a classification.
5 Classifications are agreed, but there is often a lack of clear scientific substantiation for those agreements (Nienhuis and Knegtering 2018).

Is the DSM a diagnostic or classification system?

Although the title DSM starts with diagnostic, it is "only" a classification system and therefore impersonal. The psychiatrist assesses which symptoms are present in someone and whether these symptoms meet the criteria for a particular disorder. Thus, patients with the same DSM classification do have a number of symptoms in common. However, because many combinations of symptoms are possible that lead to the same classification, the symptoms of two patients with the same DSM classification can nevertheless be very different from each other.

Are there other classification systems?

In addition to the DSM, there are also other classification systems. For example, the World Health Organization developed the International Statistical Classification of Diseases and Related Health Problems (ICD). However, these classification systems are generally not used in clinical psychiatry.

Why is there a DSM-5?

New versions of the DSM are appearing, because of advancing insights based on scientific research and changing opinions. In the DSM-5 the criteria of psychotic disorders have been changed from the fourth edition (American Psychiatric Association. 1952, 1968, 1982, 1987, 1994, 2013).

How has the classification of schizophrenia developed in the various editions of the DSM?

The DSM-II appeared in 1968. Schizophrenia was described as a condition characterized by a disturbance in thinking, mood and behavior. It was stated that thoughts may lead to misinterpretation of reality and sometimes to delusions and hallucinations. The minimum duration of these symptoms for the classification of schizophrenia was not established in the DSM-II. As a result, many psychotic disorders at the time met the classification schizophrenia. For example, if someone had unusual ideas and occasionally heard voices but actually functioned reasonably well, then they were classified as having schizophrenia at that time. Today such a problem would not meet the classification criteria of schizophrenia.

The DSM-III appeared in 1982, with specific criteria per classification for the first time. This was done in order to achieve more agreement between different psychiatrists. The DSM-III explicitly stated that the criteria were formulated on the basis of clinical judgment and that a good scientific basis was lacking. According to the DSM-III, schizophrenia should be understood as a group of disorders with possibly different causes and a different course. Therefore, the term "schizophrenic disorders" would actually be better. The criteria describe that the onset of the disorder must be before the age of 45 and that functioning must have deteriorated. In addition, the disorder must last for at least six months.

For the first time in the DSM-III the classification of schizophreniform disorder is described. In the case of a schizophreniform disorder, the symptoms meet the criteria for schizophrenia, but they last for less than six months. In addition, the classification schizoaffective disorder is added for the first time. This classification can be used if a mood disorder is present for a long time or if it precedes a psychotic period.

The DSM-IV appeared in 1994. Herein the symptom criteria of schizophrenia were expanded. Disorganization, catatonia and negative symptoms were added to hallucinations or delusions.

Finally, the DSM-5 was released in 2013. The DSM-5 strongly warns that we should not think that schizophrenia is an objective, defined disease. Consideration was given to a more dimensional approach to the disorders, but it turned out to be impossible to give a valid dimensional scheme because good research data were lacking. Another hot topic was the inclusion of a so-called "psychosis risk syndrome". Because it was feared that this unspecific condition would lead to overtreatment and stigmatization, it has not been included as an independent classification although it is described under the heading of a "residual classification". Because schizophrenia subtypes varied over time and could not be reliably identified, they are no longer included in the DSM-5. Subtypes were, for example, the paranoid subtype or the disorganized subtype (American Psychiatric Association. 1952, 1968, 1982, 1987, 1994, 2013).

A dimension scale has been added to capture the substantial variation in different symptom dimensions. This has been done because it is clear that the severity of symptoms can vary widely over time and between patients. It remains to be investigated whether this measurement scale can be reliably filled in by psychiatrists in clinical practice and whether it provides valuable information (Nienhuis and Knegtering 2018).

What are the DSM-5 criteria for classification schizophrenia and other psychotic disorders?

There are three different criteria (A., B. and C.) that must be met for the classification of schizophrenia:

A. Two or more of the following symptoms must be present (In any case, there must be one of the first three phenomena: delusions, hallucinations or disorganized speech.):

1 delusions;
2 hallucinations;
3 disorganized speech;
4 severely disorganized or catatonic behavior;
5 negative symptoms.

These symptoms must each be present a significant portion of the time for at least one month.

So, nine different combinations of two symptoms are possible: delusions and hallucinations; delusions and disorganized speech; delusions and catatonic behavior; delusions and negative symptoms; hallucinations and disorganized speech; hallucinations and catatonic behavior; hallucinations and negative symptoms; disorganized speech and catatonic behavior; disorganized speech and negative symptoms.

B. The complaints must lead to a lower level of functioning in one or more areas of life, such as work, study, social contacts or self-care.

C. The phase with active symptoms (meeting criterion A) must therefore last at least one month. In addition, symptoms of the disorder must be present for at least six months. The six months can consist of different phases:

1 the prodromal phase (precedes the clearly psychotic phase and may consist of any deterioration in functioning that occurred uninterruptedly before the psychotic phase and which appears to belong to the disease process);
2 the psychotic phase;
3 the residual phase (bothersome symptoms of the condition are still present)

(American Psychiatric Association 2013).

What kind of symptoms may be present in the prodromal and residual phase?

First of all, in the prodromal phase attenuated forms of the positive symptoms may be present. So, suspicion or ideas of grandeur without the conviction of a delusion. A persistent change in normal behavior, for example withdrawing or neglecting yourself, can also belong to the prodromal phase. In the phase after a psychosis, it may be more difficult to think clearly or concentrate, or there may be a lack of energy and flattened emotions (American Psychiatric Association 2013).

Which exclusion criteria are there?

Exclusion criteria are intended to better distinguish different classifications:

Criterion D is to rule out a "primary mood disorder". This means that if someone's complaints fit better within a depressive disorder, this classification has to be made.

Criterion E is to rule out an organic cause. For example, a psychosis that is exclusively caused by drugs or medicines, or by a physical illness. If so, you can not use the classification schizophrenia.

Criterion F is about the distinction with an autism spectrum disorder. In order to qualify as schizophrenia in someone with autism, the positive symptoms hallucinations or delusions must be clearly present (American Psychiatric Association 2013).

What are the DSM-5 criteria of the schizophreniform disorder?

For the classification schizophreniform disorder all the criteria for schizophrenia are met, but a schizophreniform disorder lasts for less than 6 months. If someone who has been classified with a schizophreniform disorder continues to experience symptoms for longer than six months, the classification will change from schizophreniform disorder to schizophrenia (American Psychiatric Association 2013).

What are favorable prognostic features in schizophreniform disorder?

If one (or more) of the following four characteristics is present, the probability of a favorable prognosis is higher:

1 The psychosis develops acutely: within four weeks after the first change in behavior.
2 There is confusion or bewilderment when psychosis is worst.
3 There was good social and professional functioning prior to the psychosis.
4 There is no flat affect [that means the emotions are vivid] (American Psychiatric Association 2013).

What are the DSM-5 criteria of the schizoaffective disorder?

This classification is intermediate between schizophrenia and a bipolar disorder:

The A criteria for schizophrenia must have been met, and more than half of the time that the disorder was present, there must have been a mood disorder (a depressive or a manic state).

There must be a period of at least two weeks during which there were psychotic symptoms without simultaneously occurrence of a disordered mood. If there are only psychotic symptoms during a mood disorder, then the classification is a bipolar disorder. So, if a person only experiences psychotic symptoms when he or she is depressed or in a manic state, then they meet the bipolar disorder classification criteria (American Psychiatric Association 2013).

What are the DSM-5 criteria for delusional disorder?

The main feature of the delusional disorder is the presence of delusions for at least one month. Beyond the problems that arise directly from the delusions, there should be no limitations in functioning. Hallucinations may be present as long as they are substantively related to the delusion and are not too prominent. The patient who meets the delusional disorder classification is able to function well in areas of life other than those to which the delusion refers. An example of this is someone who is convinced that city officials are always out to work against him. As a result of this belief, he is constantly involved in lawsuits. He is also a loving partner and good father who works to everyone's satisfaction (American Psychiatric Association 2013).

What are the DSM-5 criteria of the brief psychotic disorder?

There may be delusions, hallucinations or incoherent speech, or catatonic or confused behavior. The psychotic period lasts longer than one day, but less than one month. After that, there is a full recovery to normal functioning (American Psychiatric Association 2013).

What are the DSM-5 criteria for the psychotic disorder due to a general medical condition?

A known physical condition must be the direct cause of the hallucinations or delusions, and the consciousness is clear [otherwise you call it a delirium] and there is no serious progressive memory disorder [otherwise there may be dementia] (American Psychiatric Association 2013).

What are the DSM-5 criteria of the drug induced drug psychotic disorder?

There must be a direct link between the use of a drug or medication and the development of hallucinations or delusions. After discontinuation of the drug or medications, the psychotic symptoms should disappear completely within a few days up to a week. So, if someone continues to have psychotic symptoms after not taking drugs for a week, then there is more to it than a psychosis due to drugs (American Psychiatric Association 2013).

What are the DSM-5 criteria of catatonia?

Catatonia can manifest itself in motor symptoms (stiffening of the muscles or adopting the same posture for a long time), little speech, withdrawal behavior, (sometimes) excitement, and bizarre and repetitive behavior. Catatonia can occur in schizophrenia, but can also co-occur with anxiety disorders, mood disorders or somatic problems (American Psychiatric Association 2013).

What are the DSM-5 criteria of the "other specified schizophrenia spectrum or other psychotic disorder"?

This classification is intended for conditions that do not fit into the other boxes. It is a residual classification that is given when a psychotic state does not meet any of the other classifications of psychotic disorders. For example: someone only has delusions, but functioning is severely limited in several areas (American Psychiatric Association 2013).

What are the DSM-5 criteria of the "Unspecified Schizophrenia Spectrum or Other Psychotic Disorder"?

This classification is given if there is still insufficient clarity to be able to give another classification in the schizophrenia spectrum. For example, because the psychiatrist still knows too little about a patient who has psychotic complaints because she has only seen the patient briefly or has not yet received additional information from the family or the GP. It is a temporary classification. As soon as more is known, the classification will be changed (American Psychiatric Association 2013).

How come classifications of the same person's problems sometimes change?

Sometimes this is because a problem changes, which may justify a different classification. Sometimes this is also because information becomes available that changes the perspective on the problems. Sometimes it is because one psychiatrist or psychologist interprets the information differently. And sometimes it is because new symptoms arise or because previously existing symptoms disappear (Nienhuis and Knegtering 2018).

References

American Psychiatric Association. 1952. Diagnostic and Statistical Manual: Mental Disorders. Washington, DC: American Psychiatric Press.

American Psychiatric Association. 1968. Diagnostic and statistical manual of mental disorders (2nd ed.). Washington, DC: American Psychiatric Press.

American Psychiatric Association. 1982. Diagnostic and statistical manual of mental disorders (3rd ed.). Washington: American Psychiatric Press.

American Psychiatric Association. 1987. Diagnostic and statistical manual of mental disorders (3rd rev. ed.). Washington, DC: American Psychiatric Press.

American Psychiatric Association. 1994. Diagnostic and statistical manual of mental disorders (4th ed.). Washington, DC: American Psychiatric Press.

American Psychiatric Association. 2013. Diagnostic and statistical manual of mental disorders (5th ed.). Washington: American Psychiatric Press. American Psychiatric Association.

Nienhuis, Fokko and Knegtering, Rikus. 2018. "Classificatie van psychotische stoornissen" In Handboek schizofreniespectrumstoornissen, edited by Wiepke Cahn, Inez Myin-Germeys, Richard Bruggeman, Lieuwe de Haan. Amsterdam: De Tijdstroom.

CHAPTER 6

DIAGNOSIS OF VULNERABILITY AND RESILIENCE

Why is the classification schizophrenia not a diagnosis?

If someone is classified as having schizophrenia, it means that the psychiatric symptoms meet the criteria of the DSM-5. But that's not a personal diagnosis. In a diagnosis you also pay attention to the background, triggering and protective factors, and the impact on functioning. A diagnosis is written on the person and also gives direction to the treatment plan. Diagnosis tries to summarize what is going on, what the severity is and what course can be expected. From a personal diagnosis you arrive at the most appropriate treatment options. So, a classification only indicates that the symptoms meet certain criteria, while to really say something about a person with difficulties you need a diagnostic description.

What is described in a diagnosis?

At least the following six components are considered: classification, stage, dimensions, individual profile, triggering factors and sustaining factors. Classification was discussed in the previous chapter. In addition, a diagnosis describes the phase in which the condition is (the stage; see also below), which symptoms are present and to what degree of severity (the dimensions), and what the unique characteristics of the person are. Consider the latter's characteristics and typical behaviors, including additional psychiatric and physical problems (the profile), and the patient's circumstances, including his social environment. But the individual profile also includes a person's strengths and resilience. Triggering factors are factors that have contributed to a person becoming psychotic (for example: a breakup or cannabis use). Finally, sustaining factors contribute to the persistence of the problems (for example: homelessness or persistent drug use).

What is a stage?

The concept of stage was originally used in medicine to determine the extent and spread of a malignant tumor. A stage is a well-defined phase in a disease process. In early stages, the outlook is more favorable and treatment need to be less invasive.

Which stages are distinguished in schizophrenia spectrum disorders?

Five phases are distinguished in schizophrenia spectrum disorders:

1 Premorbid phase: a phase without obvious psychological or social problems. You actually always determine this phase afterwards.
2 Prodromal phase: a phase with the onset of mild psychotic symptoms and social problems.
3 First psychosis: a phase in which someone clearly has psychotic complaints for the first time.
4 Recurrent psychosis: a phase in which someone develops a new psychosis after being recovered from the previous psychosis.
5 Chronic psychosis: a phase in which someone suffers from a psychosis for a long time. Usually there is less good social functioning (De Haan et al. 2018).

It is certainly not the case that people go through all phases. And it is certainly not the case that once you are in the chronic phase, it can never get better. We know from research that there is a lot of switching (back and forth) between the different stages.

What is the risk that someone seeking help with mild psychotic symptoms will develop a psychotic disorder?

This question is about people who have a so-called ultra-high risk (UHR) of psychosis. A meta-analysis (see Chapter 7 for an explanation of that term) shows that this probability is about 20 percent; later studies indicate a slightly lower percentage. If people seeking help with mild psychotic symptoms also withdraw socially, the chance of developing psychosis is somewhat higher than 20 percent. For a further discussion of UHR research, see Chapter 10.

What different symptom dimensions are common in schizophrenia?

The DSM-5 includes a symptom dimension list called "Clinicians Rated Dimensions of Psychosis Symptom Severity DSM-5". It describes eight symptom dimensions relevant to psychosis: hallucinations, delusions, disorganized speech, abnormal psychomotor skills, negative symptoms, cognitive impairment, depression and mania. The severity of these symptoms can be assessed on a scale with five measuring points (from absent to very severe). It remains to be investigated whether this list really measures what it should measure and whether it can be filled in reliably by different psychiatrists. It is an improvement that more attention is now being paid to the differences in symptoms and the different degrees of severity of these symptoms (American Psychiatric Association 2013, De Haan et al. 2018).

Why are profile characteristics determined?

Profile characteristics are biological, psychological or social factors. Profile traits are chosen because they are important to a treatment plan and because they can predict the course of the disorder or response to treatment. In clinical practice you use a limited number of profile characteristics.

What is a practical set of profile characteristics (and why was this chosen)?

I compiled a list of profile characteristics on the basis of two criteria: 1] research data on the predictive value of characteristics; 2] the value of the profile characteristic for the treatment plan.

The selected profile characteristics [and the reasons for their selection] are:

*Daytime activities and social rol*e. We know from research that the chance of a new psychosis doubles when poor social functioning is present. Finding daytime activities, for example in the form of work or training, is in its own right important but may also help to prevent new psychotic episodes.

Support system. Living alone or without family involvement is associated with an increased risk of a psychosis relapse. Involving family in treatment is therefore a priority.

Physical problems. Patients with schizophrenia have a shorter life expectancy on average, mainly due to illnesses related to smoking. Substantial weight gain is also common with antipsychotic use, which increases the risk of diabetes and cardiovascular disease. Lack of exercise also plays a role. Specific attention to these risks is a priority in the treatment.

Personal recovery. Despite symptoms or limitations, patients can regain a sense of control and personal recovery. Conversely, it is possible that patients are still relatively unaffected by symptoms of the disorder, but still feel at the mercy of an uncontrollable fate. Attention to personal recovery and valuing the strength of patients is of great importance in therapy.

Substance use. Addiction greatly increases the chance that you as a patient will not adhere strictly to treatment (non-adherence to therapy), that you will develop psychosis again and that you will develop more serious positive symptoms. Addiction is also associated with a higher risk of suicide. Heavy substance use is also associated with an unfavorable social outcome. For all these reasons, reducing substance use is a top priority in the treatment plan.

Illness insight. When you have little insight into your own psychiatric problem, this increases the chance of a new psychosis, more serious symptoms and non-compliance. Having a lot of insight into your psychiatric problems is associated with fewer serious positive symptoms, but unfortunately also with more depressive symptoms. Apparently, you can get down when you realize you are vulnerable. That's understandable, especially if you don't know what to do. Illness insight sometimes appears to be difficult or impossible to improve and can be part of the disease. It is sometimes very alienating for family members when they notice that a patient really does not see that there is a psychiatric problem. On the other hand, it is also understandable from patient's point of view. If you are really convinced of something, you cannot simply be dissuaded from it. No one can rise above themselves. Interventions in people with psychosis who have no insight into illness need to prioritize to make connection, making contact and try to get concensus on a shared agenda.

Aggression. Aggression and hostility are problematic in itself and also strongly relate to problems in collaboration. Preventing the return of aggression is therefore an important treatment goal.

Suicidality. Past suicide attempts, history of suicide in the family and a recent loss of a close relative increase the likelihood of a suicide attempt. Preventing suicide attempts and suicide is an extremely important treatment goal.

Collaboration. A good relationship with the professional caregiver is particularly important: good collaboration is associated with compliance and a favorable treatment outcome. When there is good treatment alliance, most treatment goals can be achieved. Conversely, it is often extremely difficult to accomplish even minor treatment goals without collaboration.

"life events". Childhood trauma is associated with more non-adherence to therapy and a more difficult establishment of a treatment relationship. Trauma in patients with a schizophrenia spectrum disorder can often be successfully treated with psychological interventions (Alvarez-Jimenez et al. 2012; De Haan et al. 2018).

What is the value of profile characteristics in your treatment plan?

Abovementioned profile characteristics are important for developing a treatment plan. They can serve as a basis for treatment goals, for example finding daytime activities, but also indicate risks in the treatment that the patient and the therapist must take into account. If a number of unfavorable profile characteristics occur together, then they have a stronger influence on collaboration and medication adherence. For example, a combination of substance use, poor understanding of illness, aggression, and limited social inclusion increases the risk of an unfavorable course. Fortunately, you sometimes also see that a change in a certain profile characteristic also mitigates other unfavorable factors. For example, if someone gets a job, the use of drugs decreases and collaboration often improves. Improving social support can also have such an effect. In addition, a relatively large amount of research has been conducted into predictors of adherence, which almost always refers to the use of antipsychotic medication. Adherence to therapy is often worse when the following profile characteristics are present: substance dependence, poor understanding of illness, hostility, lack of social support, and poor treatment alliance (De Haan et al. 2018).

References

Alvarez-Jimenez, M., Priede, A., Hetrick, S.E., Bendall, S., Killackey, E., Parker, A.G. e.a. 2012.

Risk factors for relapse following treatment for first episode psychosis: A systematic review and meta-analysis of longitudinal studies. Schizophrenia Research, 139(1-3), 116-128.

American Psychiatric Association. 2013. Diagnostic and statistical manual of mental disorders (5th ed.). Washington: American Psychiatric Press. American Psychiatric Association.

De Haan, Lieuwe et al. 2018. “Diagnostiek naar categorie, stadium, dimensie en profiel” In Handboek schizofreniespectrumstoornissen, edited by Wiepke Cahn, Inez Myin-Germeys, Richard Bruggeman, Lieuwe de Haan. Amsterdam: De Tijdstroom.

PART 3.

SCIENTIFIC RESEARCH

CHAPTER 7

CONCEPTS IN SCIENTIFIC RESEARCH

In this chapter I explain a number of terms that are used in scientific publications.

What is Scientific Research?

Scientific research is a systematic and verifiable quest for knowledge. "Systematic" means that the research is conducted according to accepted scientific methods. "Verifiable" means that the design and method are transparent and are critically assessed by fellow scientists. The characteristic of the scientific method is that everyone can criticize the way of research and that there may and must be discussion about the advantages and disadvantages of the chosen research method, about the way in which the data have been analyzed, and about the way in which the findings have been interpreted. That is the beauty of scientific research: in essence, it is about thinking clearly and motivating your choices. Anyone who thinks clearly and logically can form an opinion about it. In principle, it does not matter how famous you are or how powerful: anyone who understands the scientific method can get involved. That's not to say everyone can always follow it. Scientists sometimes have their own language, which can be inaccessible to outsiders. But even then, the most important characteristic of science remains that people critically assess findings and that they keep looking for better methods. Often, previously widely accepted findings have to make way for newer, better or more reliable data. A good scientist is only convinced of something if the finding has proved resistant to various critical tests. And even then, she remains open to the possibility that new research may shed new light on the matter.

Unfortunately, there are problems in science. Not only fraud and conflicts of interest, but also other human characteristics can cause problems in science. For example, scientists, like others, often tend to seek confirmation for the ideas they already had. Therefore, there is a tendency among scientists to like "positive" results more than "negative", in other words: people prefer to discover that something is true than to find out that something is not true. Therefore, positive results are published more often than negative results. You call that a publication bias. The publication bias, causes a bias in our knowledge of a topic. Moreover, to know for sure, we have to repeat one and the same investigation again. But that happens too little: researchers and editors of scientific journals prefer to do something new. People find repetition boring. Scientists are just humans. But despite these problems, the built-in willingness to be critical and to accept criticism is the main virtue of the scientific method (see also Chapter 8).

What is fundamental scientific research and what is applied scientific research?

In science, a distinction is made between fundamental research and applied research. Fundamental research is aimed at understanding reality. Applied research is aimed at the application of knowledge and influencing reality.

What conditions must be met before research in humans can take place?

In research with patients, clear ethical rules apply, which must always be considered by ethical review commitees. Think of voluntary participation, guaranteeing privacy, good information, a low risk of damage, a limited burden and the extent to which the research is necessary. An independent medical ethics committee assesses patient-related research, and an investigation is only allowed if there is medical ethical approval.

Below I explain some types of research and its results. This aids in understanding scientific articles and also gives an idea of what scientists are looking for in their work.

What is a randomized trial?

In a randomized trial you can test whether a certain treatment has beneficial effects and whether there are not too many or too severe adverse effects. The treatment to be tested is applied in a group of participants (the so-called intervention group), who are compared with another group (the so-called control group). Because the effect of a treatment strongly depends on the characteristics of the person receiving the treatment, you must ensure in research that the intervention group and the control group are comparable, so that, for example, you do not unconsciously give the people with the best starting position the drug to be tested. After all, a better result of the intervention could be due to the better prognosis of the people in the intervention group. To ensure that the intervention group and the control group are as equal as possible, lots are used to determine which group you will join. This "lottery" is called randomization. The control group is treated with a placebo or another drug and sometimes they receive no treatment at all.

In the case of a study into the effect of a drug, you therefore ensure that the starting position of the people in the group that receives the drug is as close as possible to that of the group of participants who receive a "placebo" by drawing lots.

What is a double-blind study?

In addition to randomization, a scientist must also ensure that expectations or prejudices do not distort the outcome of the treatment. Therefore, blinded measurement is needed. A study with test subjects is called double blind if both the test subject and the doctor, and the researcher do not know who will receive the new treatment to be tested and who will receive the control treatment. This is done because otherwise the expectations of subjects and researchers can influence the outcome.

Expectations are very powerful. If you give someone with a convincing rationale a fake red capsule (a placebo), most people will experience pretty large effects (and side effects!). In double-blind drug studies, the new drug to be studied must look and taste exactly like the control pill or placebo. In this way, the measured difference between drug and placebo is indeed caused by the efficacy of the drug, and not caused by expectations of the patient, doctor or researcher. You call the effects that occur through trust and expectations the placebo effect.

Over the past century, double-blind research has enabled medicine to select treatments that really work. Nowadays a new drug can only be registered if it has been shown to be effective and safe in randomized controlled and blinded studies.

What is a standard deviation?

Measurements with a large group of people show dispersion or spread. "Spread" means that not everyone has the same outcome. If you want to be able to interpret the results of research, you have to take this distribution into account. For example, if you measure the temperature of a large group of sick people, you will get quite a few different results. If you graph these results, this graph resembles an old-fashioned church clock. You call this a normal distribution: very low and high values are rare, values around the mean are common (see Figure 7.1).

Figure 7.1 arow = standard deviation, 68% of the people are between mean minus standard deviation and mean plus standard deviation

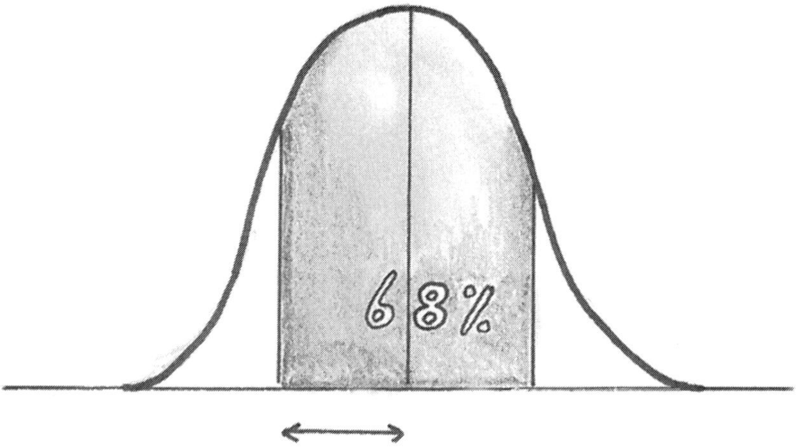

Suppose the lowest temperature that you measure in someone is 37.5 degrees, the highest 40.3 degrees. The average temperature of all participants in the study is 38.9 degrees. The spread of the different temperature measurements is important. In research, the term standard deviation is often used for this. This is a measure that expresses the spread. The mean minus one standard deviation contains about 34 percent of all participants. The mean plus one standard deviation also affects about 34 percent of people. So, 68 percent of people have a temperature that deviates a maximum of one standard deviation up or down from the mean. In this example, suppose the standard deviation is 0.7 degrees. Then 68 percent of people have a temperature between 38.2 degrees (38.9 - 0.7 = 38.2) and 39.6 degrees (38.9 + 0.7 = 39.6). See Figure 7.2 for a graphical representation of these data.

Figure 7.2 Distribution of temperature

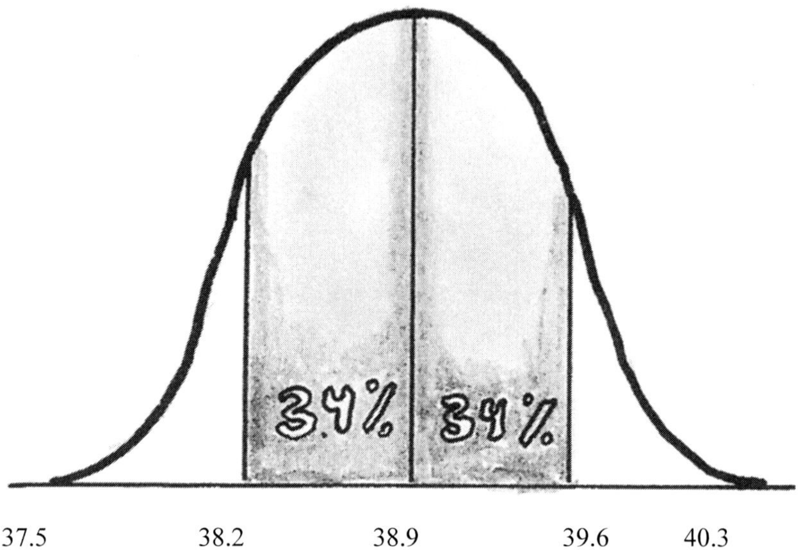

After administering the drug you want to test, you measure the temperature again. Now the lowest temperature is 36.2 degrees and the highest 39.0 degrees. The average temperature is 37.6 degrees. You can also graph these measurements and: they appear to have a normal distribution. To make things easier for ourselves, we assume that this distribution also has a standard deviation of 0.7. So now 68 percent of people have a temperature between 36.9 degrees (37.6 - 0.7 = 36.9) and 38.3 degrees (37.6 + 0.7 = 38.3).

Figure 7.3 Distribution of temperature before and after taking medication

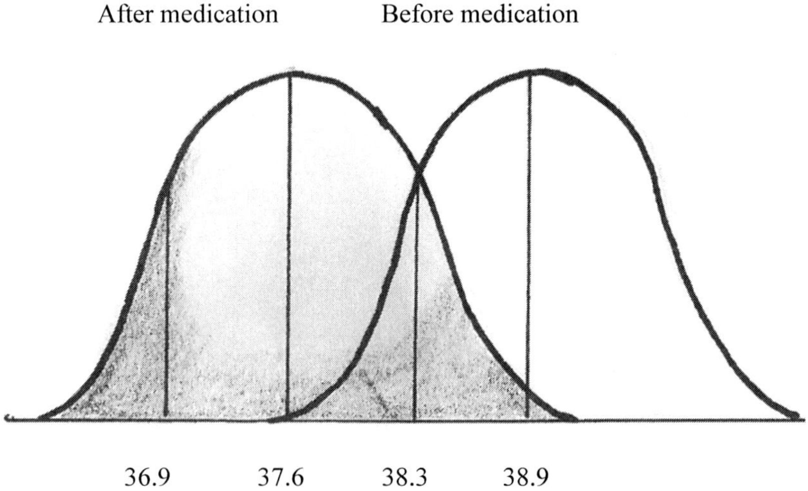

You can then also show the distribution of the difference in temperature before and after treatment with the drug in a figure. In the above example, the mean difference in temperature is: 38.9 - 37.6 = 1.3 degrees lower. The standard deviation is again 0.7. Now 68 percent of people have a temperature drop between 0.6 degrees (1.3 - 0.7 = 0.6) and 2.0 degrees (1.3 + 0.7 = 2.0). There are also some people who got a rise in temperature despite being treated with the drug: the slightest drop in temperature was negative, -0.1 degrees, which means a minimal rise. The highest temperature drop was 2.7 degrees.

Figure 7.4 Temperature drop after taking medication

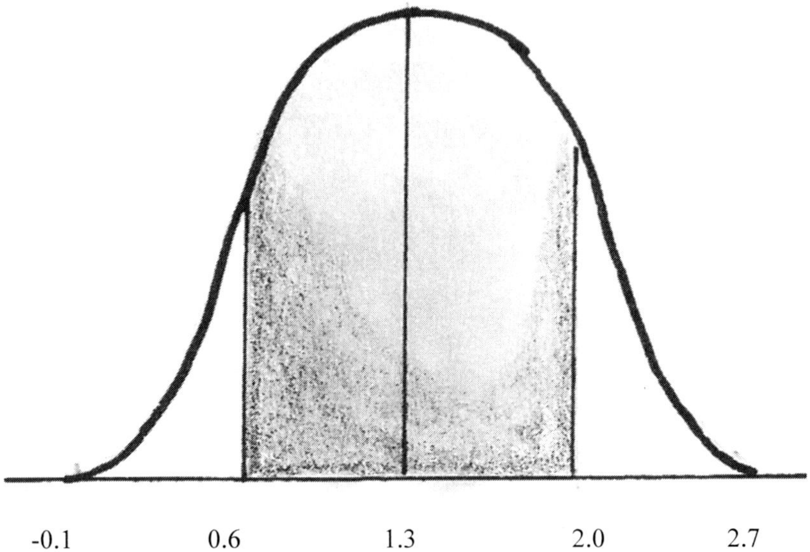

What is the effect size?

The effect size is a measure of the strength of the effect of a treatment in an intervention group compared to a control group. The effect size is calculated by dividing the difference between the mean change in the intervention and in the control condition by the standard deviation of the groups.

Let's calculate the effect size in the abovementioned example. The smallest difference between the measurement before and after administration of the drug is -0.1 degrees (this means that this person's temperature rose after taking the drug). The biggest difference was 2.7 degrees. The mean difference was 1.3 degrees. Imagine that you took the temperature in a comparable group of people before and after taking a placebo in the context of a randomized double-blind study. And now suppose that the average drop in the placebo group is 0.5 degrees, the smallest drop is -1.3 degrees (so an increase in temperature) and the largest drop is 1.9 degrees. The standard deviation is again 0.7 degrees for convenience (see Figure 7.5).

Figure 7.5 Distribution of temperature before and after placebo

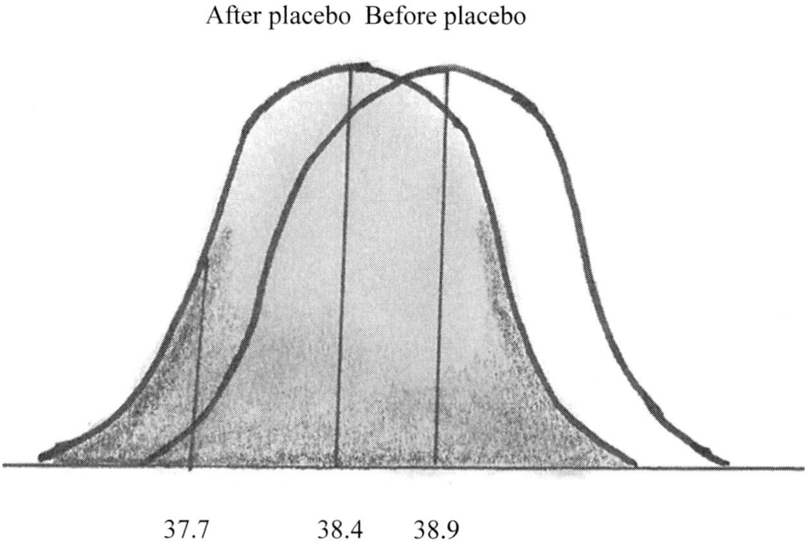

The effect size in this example is then:

(mean difference in intervention group) - (mean difference in placebo group) / (the standard deviation) = 1.3 - 0.5 / 0.7 = 1.14

Figure 7.6 Difference in temperaturedrop and effectsize after medication and after placebo

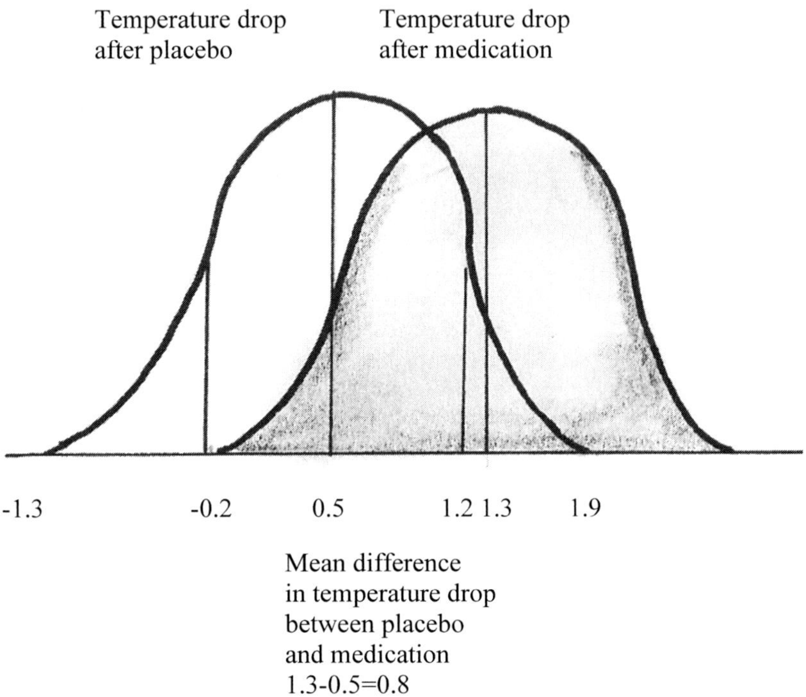

That's a big effect size! It means that the intervention shifted the sick group 1.14 standard deviation more to the favorable side than the placebo group. This means that the medicine reduces the fever significantly better than the placebo pill. This is despite the fact that not everyone keeps a fever after taking the placebo and that not everyone who receives the real medicine has a fever reduction.

The useful thing about a measure like effect size is that you can calculate it for many different studies and that way get an impression of the effect. You can therefore compare these different effect sizes. For example, the effect size of an antidepressant on mood is 0.3 and that of regular, fairly intense physical exercise on mood is also 0.3. If these effect sizes were found in comparable groups of patients, then both interventions appear to be approximately equally effective. To be more sure of this, you should do a randomized trial comparing antidepressants with physical exercise. Since you cannot do such a thing 'blindly' for the patients (after all, you know whether you took a pill or were physically active), you must ensure that at least the person who assesses the result is not aware of which intervention is given to whom. You call this a single blind study.

While an effect size of 0.3 doesn't seem like much, this is a fairly normal result in medicine and psychology. In medicine, we usually encounter effect sizes of less than about 0.5 standard deviation.

What does significance mean?

When researchers report that the outcome in the intervention group is "significantly different" from that in the placebo group, it means that the outcome is highly unlikely to be coincidental. Significance is often expressed in a so-called p-value. A p value of 0.05 means that there is a 5 percent chance that the result is a coincidence, so there is a 95 percent chance that the result is not a coincidence. But that only applies if you determined in advance that you would only research this outcome. If you measure everything that you can imagine, you can also find a significant result by chance. For example, if you perform a statistical test on a certain amount of data twenty times, the chances of finding a significant finding that are nevertheless actually coincidental are very high, perhaps as high as 100 percent. After all, twenty times a chance of 5 percent is 100 percent. That is why you should always determine in advance what you want to investigate, or what your primary outcome measure is (see the next question).

So, it's important to underline that "significance" is not the same as "important". Sometimes in large-scale research you can find very small differences that are significant. That is, while they are significant (which means that they are most likely not a coincidence), the differences are irrelevant (they don't help you much in real life). That is why a measure such as the effect size is so important: it gives you a good idea of the size of the difference or the size of the effect. For this reason, I will further mention the effect size of a therapeutic intervention, if it is known.

What is a primary outcome measure?

The primary outcome measure is the main outcome of the study. A study is set up to determine the effect on a primary outcome measure. For example, in antipsychotic research, the primary outcome measure is often "the reduction in the severity of psychotic symptoms." But a different primary outcome measure can also be chosen, for example one that is more important for the lives of patients. For example "improving the quality of life" or "improving functioning". You must therefore choose a primary outcome measure prior to each study. That is what the research is aimed at.

What does "Numbers Needed to Treat" mean?

Numbers Needed to Treat (NNT) indicates how many patients you need to treat for a given time to avoid one unfavorable outcome. NNT is the reverse of what is called the absolute risk reduction. That sounds complicated, so let's take an example. In someone with schizophrenia, the risk of a new psychotic episode in one year is 20 percent if the person takes an antipsychotic. If someone is not taking an antipsychotic, the risk of another psychotic episode is 80 percent in one year. The absolute risk reduction is then 80 - 20 = 60 percent. With that number you can then calculate the NNT:

NNT = 100 / (absolute risk reduction)

So, here: 100/60 = 1.7. This means that an average of 1.7 people have to use an antipsychotic during a year to prevent one psychotic period. That is still quite abstract. To clarify this number of 1.7 we can put it next to another example. Medicines to lower blood pressure can prevent stroke. For many of these drugs, the NNT is about 100. That is, you have to treat 100 people for a year to prevent one stroke. 99 people took the drug during that year for "nothing," but because when all 100 persons used the drug, there is one fewer stroke patient. The NNT of 1.7 for the antipsychotic is thus particularly favorable.

What does "Numbers Needed to Harm" mean?

Numbers Needed to Harm (NNH) literally means the number it takes to cause damage. NNH indicates the number of patients you need to treat to harm one patient with a particular side effect. For example, if you give two patients clozapine, one will experience sleepiness. So, the NNH in terms of sleepiness with clozapine is 2.

What is an "odds ratio"?

An odds ratio (OR) is a ratio of odds. Suppose the chance of becoming sleepy is 5 percent with a placebo. When using clozapine, this chance is much greater, namely 50 percent. Then the odds ratio for becoming sleepy with clozapine is: 50/5 = 10.

That is a very high odds ratio; in research they are usually much lower. For example, if we look at the odds ratio of developing a psychosis for someone who started smoking cannabis before the age of fifteen compared to someone who did not, then it is about 4. In concrete terms, this means roughly the following: the chance of developing any psychotic disorder over the course of your life is about 4 percent. If you then start smoking before the age of eighteen, that chance is four times 4 percent, so 16 percent.

What is a meta-analysis?

A meta-analysis is a study in which the results of previous studies are combined. This allows a more robust estimate of the effect to be given. A meta-analysis has a number of advantages:

1] Because results from different studies done in different groups of patients are taken together, the results apply to larger groups of people. Scientists say that these results are more generalizable.
2] The estimate of the actual effect is more precise.
3] Sometimes it is possible to evaluate subgroups.

There are also disadvantages. For example, sometimes the studies differ so much from each other that you compare “apples with pears”. Another possible disadvantage has to do with the available data: it often happens that studies with negative results are not published. It has already been mentioned above: we call this publication bias. If you do not take this into account, a meta-analysis will give an incorrect estimate of the effect.

What is bias?

You speak of bias when external factors have a disruptive influence on the results of an investigation, so that they do not properly reflect reality. An example is selection bias. This is the case if the researched group does not properly reflect the population about which you want to know something. Suppose you want to investigate how a drug works in schizophrenia and you only select men for the research, then there is a selection bias or gender bias in your research. Then you cannot say anything about how the drug work in all patients with schizophrenia, because the research has yielded no knowledge about women.

What is power?

Power is the probability that a certain difference will be observed significantly (see above) in the group studied. In order to find a difference that says something with some certainty about a certain group, the research must have sufficient power. The power depends on the group size, but also on the expected differences between the groups and the expected variation in results. In general, the smaller the expected difference in the primary outcome measure and the greater the spread (also known as variation) thereof, the greater the number of participants in the study must be.

What is a Correlation?

Correlation refers to the degree to which a change in one variable is associated with a similar change in another variable. Correlation is expressed as a standardized number between 1 and -1, where 1 is a perfect positive correlation, 0 is no correlation, and -1 is a perfect negative correlation. Figure 7.7 shows a number of graphs in which different correlations are shown.

Figure 7.7 Different correlations

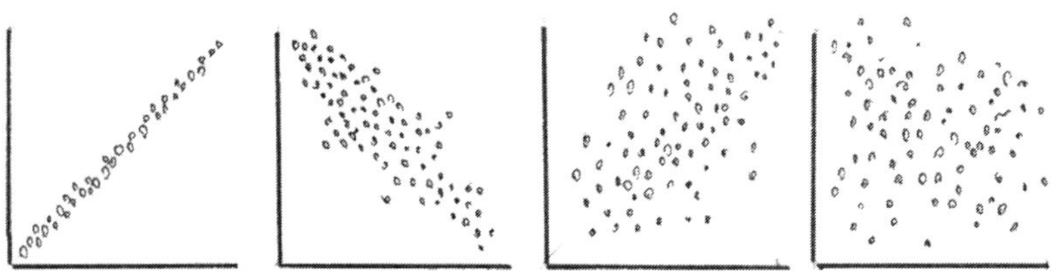

Correlation 0.9 correlation -0.7 correlation 0.5. correlation -0.3

What is a research hypothesis?

A research hypothesis is the expectation you have about the outcome before starting the research. The research hypothesis is a formulation of a possible relationship between a cause and an effect. For example: if I take pill A, the severity of the psychosis decreases more than if I take pill B. By means of research you check whether the hypothesis is correct or incorrect.

How do you determine whether a factor is most likely really a cause?

The degree to which it is probable that a certain factor is really a cause is tested on the basis of a number of criteria. These criteria are:

1 How substantial is the relationship?
2 Is the link found repeatedly in several studies?
3 How strong is the dose-response relationship? That is, if the potential causal factor increases, does the severity of the consequences also increase?
4 Does the factor precede the effect?
5 Is the relationship specific? That is to say, is the causal factor strongly related to one and the same effect and not many other consequences?
6 Could other underlying factors explain the relationship?
7 Is there a plausible explanation for the association?

The better these criteria are met, the more likely it is that the relationship found is causal.

What is validity?

Validity is the degree to which we measure what we actually want to measure. The point is whether the outcome says something about reality. Suppose you want to investigate who ever stole something in a store and you decide to investigate that by asking people the year they last stole something from a store. Then you will not receive "valid" data. You probably measure "honesty", "trust in careful handling of research data" or "absence of shame", but not the year of the last shoplifting. Your data is not valid, in other words: you do not measure what you wanted to measure. Your data do not reflect reality.

What is Reliability?

Reliability is the accuracy and precision of a measurement procedure. Reliability, for example, is about repeatability by the same researcher at different times, but also between different researchers. For example, if two researchers are taking measurements of the same object of person, you want to know whether they assess the same situation in the same way. Suppose you want to know how depressed patients are. You can find out with a measuring instrument (a kind of questionnaire) that measures the severity of someone's depression. In that case, before you start the research, you must train the researchers to administer that measuring instrument. Different investigators must arrive at the same severity score for the same patient. You call that inter-rater reliability.

CHAPTER 8

RESEARCH IN PSYCHOSIS AND SCHIZOPHRENIA

Why is scientific research on schizophrenia needed?

Because knowledge can help us find better treatments. In the past, treatments were determined by a limited number of people who enjoyed much authority. Basically, when they thought something, it was taken for granted by others. There was some debate, but it revolved around opinions. Fortunately, the situation is different now. No matter how much authority you have, you will have to provide evidence for what you claim. This scientific approach is a tremendous advance. Which of course does not mean that science has no problems. In previous chapter we discussed some of those problems. Anyway, we need more knowledge about causes, vulnerability and resilience, course, consequences, prevention and efficient and effective treatment of psychiatric disorders, and science is helping us to search for that.

What different types of schizophrenia research are there?

In the previous chapter we already described the distinction between fundamental research and applied research. Fundamental research concerns, for example, biology: genetic research, research into proteins, microorganisms and toxic substances, and into the structure and function of the brain. This research can be done in patients, but often also takes place in animals. Many people believe it is ethically right to expose animals to potentially harmful interventions or to sacrifice them in order to investigate biological processes in more detail. Sometimes this examination also takes place on deceased people. Their brain structure and microscopic variation can then be examined in detail. Fundamental research does not only concern biology, however. You can also conduct fundamental research into the development of language or aspects of social interaction. Or to certain psychological mechanisms. Other basic research is looking for data on the occurrence of psychotic disorders and schizophrenia and their causes. This type of research is called epidemiological research (see also Chapter 9).

Applied research is mainly about knowledge concerning treatment or prognosis. Usually, it concerns research into the effectiveness of an intervention with medication or psychotherapy. It may also involve research into characteristics and factors that predict a particular response to treatment.

Which different research methods are used?

Roughly speaking, research methods are divided into quantitative and qualitative research. Quantitative research involves measurements. These measurements are expressed in numbers, and they are calculated and analyzed using mathematical methods that we call statistics. Most quantitative research says something about groups. Dozens, sometimes hundreds or thousands of people have been examined. Then you get information about how things are going on average. That information does not directly say anything about an individual. An important advantage of quantitative research, however, is that you can express the result in a number and that you can compare numbers with each other.

Take, for example, the effect size, which was discussed in the previous chapter. You could even compare the effect size of a treatment with pills with that of psychotherapy. And such a comparison probably also tells you something about reality. But you have to take a lot of things into account in those kinds of comparisons. In effect studies, for example, it is first agreed what the primary outcome measure is. Suppose that is the severity of psychotic symptoms. Then you need a measuring instrument that measures the severity of psychotic symptoms. However, you can measure that in different ways. For psychotic symptoms, you can, for example, choose the measurement scale "how badly the symptom hinders someone's functioning". But who determines how much someone is bothered by a symptom? This is often the researcher who talks to the patient and his family or a nurse and assigns a grade to the severity of a symptom based on this. However, there are several different psychotic symptoms. Do you have to add up the severity of those symptoms and then take the average? And how can you be sure that one researcher measures the same as another? And if the patient feels that the symptoms are not that bothersome, but the family thinks they are, who is right? What is the real severity? With good research, all these questions have been considered, and then you can say that the outcome is reliable: you know for sure that the outcome does not depend on who measured it, and the outcome is valid: you know for sure that you measured something that is valuable in practice.

Qualitative research is about gaining insight into the way people experience certain events or phenomena. It concerns the interpretation of people, their beliefs, the meaning they attribute to certain situations. Qualitative research is about thoughts, expectations, motivations, meaning or experiences. It's about words and not about numbers. Its purpose is not to test theories, but rather to develop a theory. The researcher uses detailed interviews, asks many open questions and has less pre-defined ideas about concepts or results.

Who decides which research is carried out?

Money is needed for research. Money for the salary of researchers, for research equipment, computers and computer programs, for MRIs, laboratories, allowances for participants and so on. There are several sources for that money. It comes from general funding from universities and teaching hospitals, it comes from public and private funds, and it can come from the pharmaceutical industry. These funds can have a national, but also an international character: researchers in the Netherlands can, for example, receive European or American research funding. That money from public and private funds is generally divided based on the judgment of a group of experts. It is of course very important that this distribution is based on content and quality, and not favoritism. Usually, a fund calls for research proposals to be submitted, including an estimate of the costs. These research plans are written and submitted by the scientists involved. The best plans are selected from this. The importance of the plans, for example for solving a current problem, and their quality, for example whether the research method is correct and feasible, is considered. Fortunately, today patients and their families are increasingly involved in setting research priorities and selecting the best proposals.

What are the problems with scientific research?

Scientific research has a number of important drawbacks. We already mentioned a few in the previous chapter.

As mentioned, one of those problems comes from our tendency to want to hear a positive result. We prefer it when an association is found. It is disappointing for people when an association does not appear to exist. If something is not found, we do not find it that interesting. This tendency also influences the publication policy of scientific journals. Positive study results are more often published than negative study results. This is called publication bias. This gives us a distorted picture of reality.

Furthermore, we like to hear something new, which makes it boring to do a survey again. But repetition is desperately needed, because when we repeat research, it turns out all too often that we do not reach the same conclusions! In other words, a single study result does not say much. We need to repeat studies, only then can we be more certain about the findings.

How is it possible that there are often findings that later appear to be incorrect? That's because we tend to end up in tunnel vision. We love positive findings so much that we overemphasize supporting evidence and ignore contrary findings or clues. In addition, researchers feel pressure to publish. They would like to contribute or they like to become famous. Therefore, they tend to always find something in the data that emerged from their research. However, these are by no means always strong relationships, and there is a chance that these findings will emerge because of bias. Sometimes it is worse. There are also examples of scientific misconduct: data that has been falsified and results that have been selectively presented, for example.

It is important that science finds solutions to these problems. A step forward would be: publish negative studies more easily: studies in which the desired correlation is not found. But also: carefully repeat studies more often to test important findings, look for robust effects, and not automatically think that something is important if it is significant. Something is only important if the effect size is large enough. It would also be an important step forward if more attention were paid to the reliability of measurements. Finally, it would be very helpful if studies could only be published if a plan with a primary outcome measure was pre-approved.

What are the problems of schizophrenia research?

Scientific research into schizophrenia suffers from the above general problems. But it also has a number of specific problems. First, the definition of the classification schizophrenia is clear and reliable, but we are not sure whether we have classified something real, something valid. After all, there is a huge variation in symptoms between patients and over time. These differences mean that the averages we find in research sometimes do not say much. Certainly not about an individual patient. Many studies are also relatively small. This is because it is quite difficult to involve patients with schizophrenia in long-term scientific research.

Why are registry studies of antipsychotics meaningful?

A registry study examines routinely collected data from a large group of people included in a registry. In a randomized trial, only people who want to cooperate are examined. As a result, you miss people in such research who do not want to cooperate, for example because they are too suspicious or do not like researchers or professional caregivers. It is therefore unclear whether the outcomes of randomized trials do apply to all types of patients. In contrast, everyone was included in research within registers. The disadvantage is that you can only research very global outcome measures. The Scandinavian countries have very good registers, and much of this type of research comes from those countries. For example, registry studies from Finland have shown that the risk of re-admission is lowest if people with schizophrenia use clozapine or antipsychotics in depot form. Furthermore, such research showed that people who are treated with antipsychotics die less often prematurely than people who are not prescribed antipsychotics.

PART 4.

EPIDEMIOLOGY AND COURSE

CHAPTER 9

EPIDEMIOLOGY OF SCHIZOPHRENIA SPECTRUM DISORDERS

What is Epidemiology?

Epidemiology is the study of the occurrence and distribution of diseases in the population. An epidemiologist tries to find out how many people are affected by a disease and which causal or protective factors influence the development of the disease. In addition, an epidemiologist examines the course of a disease and tries to find out which factors influence the course.

What is the incidence of schizophrenia?

The incidence is a number that indicates how many people in the population develop a disease for the first time during a certain period (often a year).

Various overview studies have shown that the average incidence of schizophrenia is about 17 per 100,000 inhabitants per year. An important outcome of these studies is that the incidence can vary considerably per area. In some regions the incidence is only 7 new patients per 100,000 inhabitants per year, in others more than six times as high: 43 new patients per 100,000 inhabitants per year.

Which factors influence the incidence?

The incidence is much higher in large cities than in the countryside. The incidence in migrant groups also appears to be much higher: as much as 60 per 100,000. In men, the incidence was highest between the ages of 20 and 29. In women there was a less pronounced age related peak in incidence (Jablensky et al. 1992).

Figure 9.1 Incidence of schizophrenia

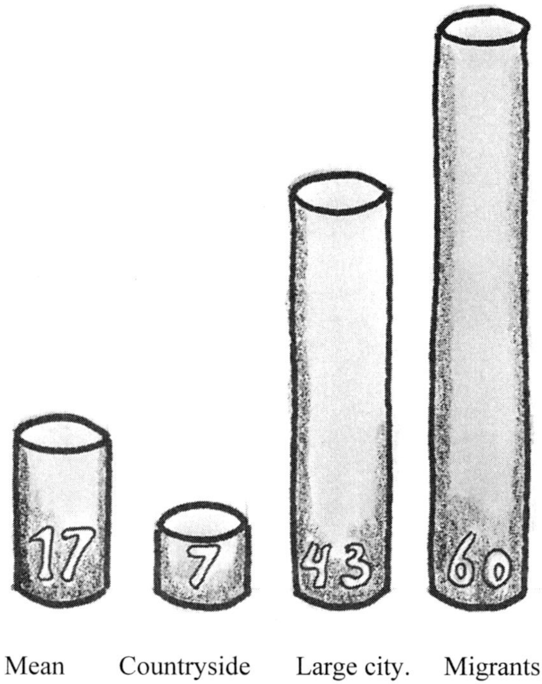

What is the prevalence of schizophrenia?

Prevalence is a number that expresses how many people in the population have or have ever had a disease at any given time. If you examine who has the disease at any given time, you are looking for the "point prevalence". "Lifetime prevalence" is the proportion of people living at that time who have had the disease at some point in their lifetime.

A recent review shows that the lifetime prevalence of schizophrenia is between 0.4 percent and 0.5 percent. That is lower than the figure stated in many books. Before, it was thought that the lifetime prevalence lied between 0.7 percent to 1 percent.

Which factors influence lifetime prevalence?

Lifetime prevalence is lower in lower-income countries. Among migrants it is almost twice as high as in the native population. This is a less striking difference than was found for the incidence: the incidence among migrants is more than three times as high.

The degree of urbanization of the environment has no clear influence on the lifetime prevalence. That is special, because the degree of urbanization has a lot of influence on the incidence, as mentioned.

What is the lifetime prevalence of other schizophrenia spectrum disorders?

Fewer studies have been conducted into the prevalence of other schizophrenia spectrum disorders than into the prevalence of schizophrenia. It is estimated that about 4 percent of the population meets the criteria for a schizophrenia spectrum disorder at some point in their lifetime. About 0.5 percent ever meet the criteria for schizophrenia and 3.5 percent ever meet the criteria for another schizophrenia spectrum disorder. In addition, it is estimated that about 3 percent of the population ever has psychotic symptoms without any obvious discomfort and without the need for help. That means that 7 percent of people ever have psychotic symptoms. Not super rare.

What is the course of schizophrenia and other schizophrenia spectrum disorders?

The course of schizophrenia and other schizophrenia spectrum disorders differs enormously.

Overall, it can be said that after about five years nearly 50 percent of patients with schizophrenia spectrum disorder have recovered. If one only looks at the course of people with schizophrenia, about 27 percent will have recovered after five years.

Furthermore, long-term studies of people with schizophrenia [who were 22-37 at the start of the study] found disease recovery in 46 to 62 percent, and social recovery in 21 to 68 percent. What is striking here is the wide variation in outcomes, but also that more than half of the patients with schizophrenia reach symptomatic recovery in the long term (Cahn et al. 2018).

How often do people with schizophrenia who have recovered from their first psychotic period have a second psychotic period?

About 70 to 80 percent of people who are no longer taking antipsychotics will have a second psychotic episode. If people do continue to use antipsychotics, the recurrence rate is still 20 to 30 percent. On the other hand, about 20 percent of people who have ever met the classification criteria for schizophrenia never experience another psychotic period, even if they are no longer taking antipsychotics. It is very important to find out who these people are. After all, they no longer need antipsychotics after their initial psychosis has passed. This question, among other things, is being investigated in the Dutch HAMLETT study that has been ongoing since 2019. HAMLETT stands for "Handling Antipsychotic Medication: Long-term Evaluation of Targeted Treatment". Several other studies around the world also try to answer the question which patients can safely discontinue their antipsychotics (for instance the RADAR study).

Which factors influence the course?

It was found that patients who continued to use cannabis developed more psychotic episodes, had more psychotic complaints and had worse social functioning after three years. Furthermore, the severity of depressive symptoms at the first measurement was associated with an unfavorable quality of life after three years. A higher verbal IQ was associated with a more favorable course, while poor memory was associated with less recovery from symptoms and more psychotic episodes (Menezes, Arenovich, and Zipursky 2006, De Nijs et al. 2014, Van der Meer et al. 2015)

How many people with schizophrenia still need care five to ten years after a first psychosis?

Overall, 20 percent of people with schizophrenia have recovered five to ten years after a first psychosis, without needing help. About 60 percent of them need outpatient care and about 20 percent require intensive outpatient or inpatient care (Wiersma et al. 1989).

How do people with schizophrenia live five to ten years after a first psychosis?

About 90 percent of people with schizophrenia live independently or with friends or family five to ten years after a first psychosis, about 6 percent live in a sheltered housing project and about 4 percent are admitted to a psychiatric hospital (Wiersma et al. 1989).

In short, what is striking in the results of research into the course of people with the classification schizophrenia?

What is striking in the research into the course of schizophrenia is that there are large differences in the degree of recovery between patients.

References

Cahn Wiepke, Slooff Cees, Wiersma Durk. 2018. "Epidemiologie en beloop" In Handboek schizofreniespectrumstoornissen, edited by Wiepke Cahn, Inez Myin-Germeys, Richard Bruggeman, Lieuwe de Haan. Amsterdam: De Tijdstroom.

Jablensky, A., Sartorius, N., Ernberg, G., e.a. (1992). Schizophrenia: manifestations, incidence and course in different cultures. A World Health Organization ten-country study. Psychol Med Monograph Supplement, 20, 1-97.

Meer, F.J. van der, Velthorst, E.; Genetic Risk and Outcome of Psychosis (group) Investigators (2015). Course of cannabis use and clinical outcome in patients with non-affective psychosis: a 3-year follow-up study. Psychol Med, 45(9), 1977-1988.

Menezes, N.M., Arenovich, T., & Zipursky, R.B. (2006). A systematic review of longitudinal outcome studies of first- episode psychosis. Psychol Med, 36, 1349-1362.

Nijs, J. de, Zoun, K., & group Investigators (2014). The association between cognitive deficits and different outcomes of schizophrenia. Psychiatr Pol, 48(6), 1087-1104.

Wiersma, D., Nienhuis, F.J., Slooff, C.J., & Giel, R. (1998). Natural course of schizophrenic disorders: A 15-year follow-up of a Dutch incidence cohort. Schizophr Bull, 24, 75-85.

CHAPTER 10

INCREASED RISK

Are there any signs indicating a high risk to develop psychosis?

In the period leading up to a first psychosis, a person may have mild, fleeting, psychosis-like experiences. These mild psychosis symptoms often occur in combination with symptoms of anxiety or depression. But not all people who have psychosis-like symptoms also develop psychosis. People with such symptoms run a higher risk of developing psychosis. If their symptoms meet certain criteria, they are also referred to as "ultra-high risk" or UHR (Boonstra et al. 2018).

How is the state of ultra high risk of developing psychosis defined?

Patrick McGorry and Alison Yung, two Australian researchers, have proposed identifying and tracking the UHR group and offering these people treatment to prevent the development of psychosis. They distinguish three groups who, if they have a marked decline in functioning, have an increased vulnerability to developing psychosis:

1. A group with mild psychotic symptoms that do not last long enough or are not severe enough to meet the criteria of a psychotic disorder (for example, they may be hallucinating once a month);
2. A group with marked psychotic symptoms lasting less than a week and disappearing completely without treatment;
3. A group with a first-degree relative (parent, brother or sister) with a schizophrenia spectrum disorder (Yung et al. 2005).

In which age group is the risk increased?

Three quarters of all psychiatric disorders manifest themselves before the age of 25. The risk of developing a psychotic disorder after the age of 35 is relatively small. However, it does happen regularly that women develop a first psychosis at the beginning of the menopause. Nevertheless, it has been decided to limit the detection of UHR to people between the ages of 14 and 35 (Fusar-Poli et al. 2012, Boonstra et al. 2018).

What is the course for people who meet the UHR criteria?

There is also a lot of variation in outcome for people in the UHR group. Overall, the mild symptoms disappear over the course of two years in more than a third of people with a UHR. We know the following from a meta-analysis: mild psychotic symptoms persist in just under 10 percent, 18 percent have developed psychosis after one year and 36 percent after three years. After that, there are hardly any more people from the UHR group who still develop psychosis. In recent years the risk of developing psychosis in UHR groups has decreased, but this is probably because people with less serious problems are now included in the UHR group. The risk of psychosis if you meet UHR criteria now varies on average between 10 and 20 percent. That is quite a risk, but attempts are being made to find groups that run an even greater risk. After all, the higher the risk, the more meaningful treatment is.

About 75 percent of people in the UHR group who eventually develop psychosis eventually meet the classification criteria of a schizophrenia spectrum disorder. About 25 percent of this group develop psychosis that fits the classification of bipolar disorder. The majority of people who meet the UHR criteria have problems with their functioning for a longer period of time (Fusar-Poli et al. 2013, Boonstra et al. 2018).

Is there a questionnaire that can be used to screen if someone might be at an ultra high risk of developing psychosis?

A questionnaire that is used to quickly determine whether someone may be at an ultra high risk of psychosis is the Prodromal Questionnaire. This questionnaire can be used when someone is referred to mental health care. The Prodromal Questionnaire contains sixteen statements, such as: "I often feel that others are doing me harm" and "I sometimes get confused about whether something I experienced was real or fantasy". After completing the questionnaire, the total score is calculated by adding up all statements answered "agree". This gives a score between 0 and 16. With a score of 6 or higher, it may be wise to further investigate whether someone meets the UHR criteria (Ising et al. 2015).

What tests can be done to determine if someone meets UHR criteria?

Follow-up research can be done with the Comprehensive Assessment of At Risk Mental State (CAARMS). With the CAARMS, special experiences that someone has are explored: how often do they occur, how severe are they and how long do the special experiences last? And what does someone think about it? Based on the outcome of the CAARMS and an assessment of social functioning, it is determined whether there is an ultra high risk of developing psychosis (Boonstra et al. 2018).

Which psychotherapeutic treatment will help prevent the risk of developing psychosis in someone at high risk?

A specific form of cognitive behavioral therapy has been developed to reduce the risk of psychosis in people in the risk group. Someone with an increased risk still has doubts about the meaning of the special experiences and then it can help to provide information, for example about the influence of dopamine. "Stress makes your dopamine system hypersensitive, which keeps you on your toes." This allows you to better understand psychosis-like experiences, worry less and reduce tension.

It also helps to experience through exercise how your tendency to watch for danger affects your fear or worry.

In addition, addiction is treated, but also anxiety and depression. Retaining work or education is of great importance. In general, the more you feel included in a group of friends, the more satisfied you are with your daily activities and the less drugs you use, the less likely you are to become unbalanced. The effects of psychotherapy on the transiationrate to psychosis are debated (Fusar-Poli et al. 2013).

Do antipsychotics have a role in the treatment in the UHR phase?

Treatment with antipsychotics in the UHR phase is not recommended. The balance between effect and side effects of antipsychotics is unfavorable in the UHR phase, and it is also impossible to predict for how long you will have to use antipsychotics. In addition, the risk of developing psychosis for someone with a UHR is an average of 10 to 20 percent per year. That is far too low to prescribe preventive antipsychotics (Fusar-Poli et al. 2013).

References

Boonstra, Nynke, Pijnenborg, Marieke, Klaassen, Rianne. 2018. "Verhoogd risico en de ultrahoogrisicofase" In Handboek schizofreniespectrumstoornissen, edited by Wiepke Cahn, Inez Myin-Germeys, Richard Bruggeman, Lieuwe de Haan. Amsterdam: De Tijdstroom.

Fusar-Poli, P., Bonoldi, I., Yung, A.R., Borgwardt, S., Kempton, M.J., Valmaggia, L., e.a., (2012). Predicting psychosis: Meta-analysis of transition outcomes in individuals at high clinical risk. *Archives of General Psychiatry*, *69(3)*, 220-229.

Fusar-Poli, P., Borgwardt, S., Bechdolf, A., Addington, J., Riecher-Rossler, A., Schultze-Lutter, F., e.a. (2013). The psychosis high-risk state: a comprehensive state-of-the-art review. *JAMA Psychiatry*, *70(1),* 107-120.

Ising, H.K., Veling, W., Loewy, R.L., Rietveld, M.W., Rietdijk, J., Dragt, S., e.a. (2012). The validity of the 16-item version of the prodromal questionnaire (pq-16) to screen for ultrahigh risk of developing psychosis in the general help-seeking population. *Schizophrenia Bulletin*, *38(6),* 1288-1296.

Yung, A.R., Yuen, H.P., McGorry, P.D., Phillips, L.J., Kelly, D., Dell'Olio, M., e.a. (2005). Mapping the onset of psychosis: the comprehensive assessment of at-risk mental states. *Australian and New Zealand Journal of Psychiatry, 39(11-12),* 964-971.

CHAPTER 11

(VERY) EARLY ONSET SCHIZOPHRENIA IN CHILDHOOD

What is very early onset schizophrenia?

When a child meets the schizophrenia classification for the first time before the age of thirteen.

What is early onset schizophrenia?

When a young person meets the schizophrenia classification for the first time between the ages of thirteenth and eighteenth. This is slightly more common, but usually people are over eighteen when they first meet the classification of schizophrenia.

How often does (very) early-onset schizophrenia occur?

The figures vary per study. A rough estimate is that less than 1 percent of patients with schizophrenia manifest themselves before the age of 10 and about 4 percent of them before the age of eighteen. On the other hand, just a little bit latter onset occurs more frequently. There are also studies showing that about 40 percent of boys who ever get the classification schizophrenia and 20 percent of girls already meet the classification at the age of nineteen (Kelleher et al. 2012, Hillegers et al. 2018).

How common are mild psychotic symptoms in children and adolescents?

Mild psychotic symptoms that cause little or no discomfort occur in 17 percent of children (between nine and twelve years) and in 7.5 percent of adolescents (between thirteen and eighteen years). Most psychotic experiences during childhood are transient.

The prevalence of mild psychotic symptoms decreases with age, while psychotic disorders increase in adolescence. The mild psychotic symptoms at a very young age have a certain overlap with the great fantasy world of young children (Hillegers et al. 2018).

Is there a greater hereditary vulnerability in (very) early onset schizophrenia?

Parents and siblings of children with (very) early-onset schizophrenia are more likely (25 percent) to have a disorder in the schizophrenic spectrum themselves than parents and siblings of someone whose schizophrenia manifested itself in adulthood (approx. 10 percent). Very early onset schizophrenia therefore has a larger hereditary component (Hillegers et al. 2018).

Is normal puberty imbalance related to the risk of developing schizophrenia?

Characteristic of normal puberty is that children are unbalanced, can have a fluctuating mood, be less motivated and can be difficult to communicate with. This imbalance is normal and is not associated with a risk of developing a psychotic illness.

Are there already abnormalities in (very) early onset schizophrenia in the phase prior to the onset of psychosis?

Problems in the development of language, motor skills, social skills and cognitive function are more common in children who show psychotic symptoms at an early age. These abnormalities are especially common in boys. Therefore, it is thought that children who become psychotic at an early age have a more severe disruption of brain development, possibly associated with greater genetic vulnerability. Delayed language development is found in 30 to 40 percent of children with (very) early onset schizophrenia. Motor development is delayed in about 50 percent of these children. Particularly characteristic is poorer social functioning: it occurs in 80 to 90 percent of them. Impulsivity and strange beliefs or perceptions are found in 30 to 80 percent of children prior to psychosis. Research in which children were followed showed that about two years before the onset of psychosis, intelligence declines. After that, the intelligence level remains stable. On average, children with (very) early-onset schizophrenia have an IQ of about 80 to 85. Related to the above problems, there are often learning difficulties, which usually require special education.

Can you prevent early onset of psychosis?

In retrospect, parents often say that their psychotic adolescent or young adult children were also previously lonely or even difficult to get along with. They had unusual fears and fantasies, and were socially withdrawn and vulnerable. So, you may wonder whether early treatment can prevent psychosis. However, there are no interventions that have been shown to prevent psychotic development in children with the above problems. The only thing that is certain is that it is unwise for children with such difficulties to start smoking cannabis.

What are the symptoms and how is the course of (very) early-onset schizophrenia?

Usually, the problems gradually start with underachievement at school, poor personal care, low energy, socially withdrawn behavior and disorganization. However, because the development was often difficult before and because it can take a while for psychotic symptoms to develop, it often takes a long time before the diagnosis is made. Frequently, children who later meet the classification of (very) early-onset schizophrenia are first diagnosed with another diagnosis, such as autism. Flat and maladjusted emotions occur in about 85 percent of children with (very) early-onset schizophrenia, lack of motivation in about 70 percent, and reduced speech in about 60 percent. The content of psychotic phenomena suits the stage of life of children (monsters, but also paranoid delusions). Visual and sensory hallucinations are more common than in adult-onset schizophrenia. Children with (very) early onset schizophrenia recover less well from a psychotic period than patients whose problems occur later. The chance of the psychosis completely disappearing is only 10 percent in children with very early onset schizophrenia. The chance that children with a psychosis will have to be re-admitted in the first years is about 80 percent. Partly because children with (very) early onset schizophrenia have early school breaks, they often remain dependent on others. Intensive support is often required at home and in special education (Hillegers et al. 2018).

Which characteristics predict an unfavorable course?

A systematic review article focusing on research into children whose disease started at an average age of 14.5 years shows that an unfavorable course is associated with a long duration of untreated psychosis and poor functioning prior to psychosis. If the psychosis suddenly starts with delusions and hallucinations in children, the prognosis is better. If the family cannot support properly or if there are major difficulties in the family, the prognosis is less favorable (Kelleher et al. 2012).

What should be considered when treating children with antipsychotics?

First, children need even lower doses of antipsychotics than adults. This is because children are more likely to have higher blood levels of antipsychotics. Furthermore, the dose should be low because children are more susceptible to parkinsonism (such as tremors and stiffness) and other movement disorders. In addition, children are also more likely to gain weight and are prone to develop a "metabolic syndrome". Metabolic syndrome refers to the following characteristics: substantial fat accumulation around the abdomen; cholesterol abnormalities in the blood; a higher blood sugar level; and high blood pressure.

This can have major long-term health consequences for children (Harvey, James and Shields 2016). In addition, children are also more sensitive to a high level of "prolactin", which can occur as a side effect of antipsychotics. A high level of prolactin can disrupt hormonal development, growth and puberty development and increases the risk of osteoporosis. This is especially a problem during risperidone treatment. The pharmaceutical company has done a lot of research into risperidone treatment in children. These studies show that risperidone has a good antipsychotic effect and that the side effects are not too bad in the short term. For this reason, risperidone is often prescribed by child and adolescent psychiatrists. After all, it has been studied in children and adolescents. But risperidone contains a breakdown product, which does not enter the brain itself, but which causes dopamine receptors outside the brain to be blocked (Kelleher et al., 2012). As a result, the blockade of dopamine receptors in the pituitary gland becomes high, causing the prolactin level to rise sharply. So, despite the fact that risperidone has been widely researched in children and although it has no more side effects in the short term than other drugs, it has adverse effects in the long term and in my opinion it should preferably not be prescribed to children and adolescents.

References

Harvey, R.C., James, A.C., & Shields, G.E. (2016). A systematic review and network meta-analysis to assess the relatively efficacy of antipsychotics for the treatment of positive and negative symptoms in early-onset schizophrenia. CNS Drugs, 30(1), 27-39.

Hillegers, Manon, Bolhuis, Koen, Scheepers, Floortje. 2018. "Kinderpsychose" In Handboek schizofreniespectrumstoornissen, edited by Wiepke Cahn,

Inez Myin-Germeys, Richard Bruggeman, Lieuwe de Haan. Amsterdam: De Tijdstroom.

Kelleher, I., Connor, D., Clarke, M.C., Devlin, N., Harley, M., & Cannon, M. (2012). Prevalence of psychotic symptoms in childhood and adolescence: a systematic review and meta-analysis of population-based studies. Psychol Med, 42(9), 1857-1863.

CHAPTER 12

SCHIZOPHRENIA DEVELOPING LATER IN LIFE

What is late onset schizophrenia?

When symptoms of schizophrenia first appear after the age of 40.

What is very late onset schizophrenia?

When symptoms of schizophrenia first occur after the age of 60 years. There are psychiatrists who think that it is not correct to classify the group of patients whose symptoms only develop so late in the category schizophrenia. This is because in people who meet the classification criteria so late in life for the first time, negative symptoms are rare and the degree of disorganization is limited. Assigning the classification schizophrenia in these cases, does not fit the idea of schizophrenia as a developmental disorder. Nevertheless, it is clear that serious psychotic disorders can also occur for the first time after the age of 60, without the presence of dementia or a mood disorder. In addition, these conditions meet the classification criteria for schizophrenia (Meesters 2018).

How often does (very) late-onset schizophrenia occur?

It is not entirely clear how often (very) late onset schizophrenia occurs. There are several estimates: In 23 to 29 percent of patients with schizophrenia, symptoms would manifest for the first time after the age of 40. However, there are major differences between men and women. According to a recent meta-analysis, nearly 40 percent of women whose problems qualify for the classification as schizophrenia are diagnosed for the first time after the age of 40, while less than 20 percent of men are for the first time diagnosed after the age of 40. A first diagnosis after the age of 60 is made in about 19 percent of women, compared to only 7 percent of men. What this shows in any case is that it is by no means rare for problems classified as schizophrenia to manifest itself for the first time at a later age (Meesters 2018).

Do the symptoms differ in (very) early-onset schizophrenia and (very) late-onset schizophrenia?

There are some striking differences between symptoms in (very) early-onset schizophrenia and (very) late-onset schizophrenia. Delusions often have a haunting character in people with (very) late onset schizophrenia. It is remarkable that patients with very late onset schizophrenia are often convinced that walls or ceilings are pervious to people, animals or materials (Cohen, Meesters and Zhao 2015).

In (very) late onset schizophrenia, hallucinations relatively often involve images, feelings or smell in addition to sound. Disorganization is less common in late onset schizophrenia and is almost always absent in very late onset schizophrenia. Negative symptoms are rare, especially in late onset schizophrenia. Perhaps negative symptoms are mainly associated with a developmental disorder that starts at an early age (Meesters 2018).

What is the course of cognitive function in (very) late onset schizophrenia?

Studies into the development of cognitive function in late-onset or very late-onset schizophrenia yield different results. However, the profile of cognitive dysfunction is not very different from that of early-onset schizophrenia. In the short term, the course of cognitive dysfunctions appears to be stable. A number of studies did find a slightly increased risk of dementia in older patients with schizophrenia (Cohen, Meesters and Zhao 2015, Meesters 2018).

Why is it that a relatively large number of women develop a first psychosis at a later age?

A relatively large number of women develop a first psychosis at a later age. The theory is that during menopause, estrogen levels drop, revealing an underlying vulnerability. There are also other findings that indicate the protective effect of estrogens. During the menstrual cycle, the severity of psychosis increases when estrogen levels fall. Another finding that points to the beneficial effects of estrogens is the fact that randomized double-blind studies of the effects of administered estrogens show that they have antipsychotic effects. Finally, another factor that may play a role in the underrepresentation of women in the younger age group is that women are less likely than men to display maladaptive or aggressive behavior. This could mean that in women there is a more substantial risk that a psychotic condition goes unreckognized (Meesters 2018).

Are there already problems with functioning before the psychosis appears in patients with (very) late onset schizophrenia?

A number of studies report that patients with very late onset schizophrenia were more likely to have a withdrawn life and already had magical ideas or were somewhat suspicious prior to the psychosis. Social isolation prior to psychosis is common (Meesters 2018).

Do problems with hearing and vision precede (very) late onset schizophrenia?

Hearing impairment is associated with a greater likelihood of becoming suspicious. Impaired vision could also be a triggering or causal factor. However, both have not yet been properly researched (Cohen, Meesters and Zhao 2015).

Is migration a risk factor for (very) late onset schizophrenia?

Migration as a risk factor for (very) late onset schizophrenia has been studied in London. African and Caribbean migrants had more often (very) late onset schizophrenia. This was not the case for migrants from Bangladesh, who are generally more integrated into English society. On average, these migrants had lived in London for thirty years (Brodaty 2003).

Have specific neurobiological abnormalities been found in (very) late onset schizophrenia?

When it comes to neurological abnormalities specific to (very) late-onset schizophrenia, the findings vary from study to study. The variation mainly shows that within this group of patients there are at least as large differences as between patients with earlier developed schizophrenia (Meesters 2018).

What other conditions can cause symptoms similar to those of (very) late onset schizophrenia?

When psychotic symptoms first appear in old age, they are more likely to be caused by a physical condition than at a young age. We will briefly discuss two conditions with a physical cause: delirium and dementia.

Someone with delirium can have psychotic symptoms. In delirium, a physical cause, such as an infection or intoxication, causes impaired brain function. The consciousness in those cases varies: people sometimes have a less clear consciousness.

Someone with dementia can also be psychotic. Dementia is characterized by the deterioration of brain function due to increasing damage to the brain. People with dementia do have a clear consciousness, but usually suffer from gradually increasing memory disorder.

Psychotic symptoms can also occur with another psychiatric problem, such as depression. This usually involves an increasingly serious depressed mood before the psychotic symptoms develop.

Is the treatment of (very) late onset schizophrenia different?

Psychotherapeutic treatment can help the elderly as well as the young.

Regarding the treatment with antipsychotics, adjustments are necessary when schizophrenia develops late in life. In general, the content of delusions in the elderly is tough. Antipsychotics can help reduce anxiety, but usually the psychotic beliefs do not disappear completely. Antipsychotics should be taken in lower doses because older people break down and excrete drugs to a lesser extent. Furthermore, elderly patients are more likely to suffer from parkinsonism as a side effect, such as stiffness or tremors. Therefore, a dosage is often required that is between 25 and 75 percent of what is usual in adults. In addition, elderly patients are more prone to dizziness, balance disorders, difficulties with vision and urination problems. Some antipsychotics have these so-called “anticholinergic” side effects to a great extent. Therefore, these antipsychotics should either not be given or used in very low doses (see also Chapter 41 on antipsychotics).

Older people who have been taking antipsychotics for many years may sometimes experience more side effects, or other side effects than before. This may be because the breakdown and excretion of drugs decrease with age. It is important to then adjust the dosage or the drug (Cohen, Meesters and Zhao 2015).

References

Brodaty, H., Sachdev, P., Koschera, A., Monk, D., & Cullen, B. (2003). Long-term outcome of lateonset schizophrenia: 5-Year follow-up study. British Journal of Psychiatry, 183, 213-219.

Cohen, C.I., Meesters, P.D., & Zhao, J. (2015). New perspectives on schizophrenia in later life: implications for treatment, policy, and research. The Lancet Psychiatry, 2(4), 340-350.

Meesters, Paul David. 2018. "Late-onset schizofrenie" In Handboek schizofreniespectrumstoornissen, edited by Wiepke Cahn, Inez Myin-Germeys, Richard Bruggeman, Lieuwe de Haan. Amsterdam: De Tijdstroom.

CHAPTER 13

(SOCIAL) COGNITIVE PROBLEMS

What is Cognition?

Cognition is the ability to absorb and process information so that it contributes to knowledge. The heading "cognition" covers various cognitive processes or functions, such as attention, perception, memory, language, reasoning or decision making.

What is Social Cognition?

Social cognition consists of cognitive processes, as described above, that are involved in understanding social situations and understanding other people. Through social cognition we understand the behavior of other people and we can communicate effectively with each other.

What Are Cognitive Symptoms?

These are problems with or changes in your cognitive function. For example, a reduced ability to concentrate or keep your attention, problems with planning and keeping an overview or memory problems. Sometimes a person also has problems assessing social information quickly and correctly, such as a facial expression or the tone of a voice.

Which cognitive domains are distinguished?

Three domains of cognitive functioning are distinguished:

1] neurocognition, which includes basic functions such as attention and memory;
2] social cognition, which includes mental processes that play a role in social contact; and
3] metacognition, this includes thinking about one's own thinking.

In the following I discuss questions about these domains.

Neurocognition

Which basic cognitive functions differ on average in people with schizophrenia spectrum disorder from people without schizophrenia?

In some of the people with a schizophrenia spectrum disorder, abnormalities are found in the following cognitive functions:

1] speed of information processing;
2] attention;
3] working memory;
4] declarative memory; and
5] executive functions.

Speed of information processing is about the speed at which someone carries out cognitive processes. This is an important basic function. For example, it is about how quickly you perceive changes or how quickly you can respond. Many other cognitive functions depend on the information processing speed. If you process information less quickly, you may already be confronted with new information while you are still processing the old information. You can imagine that something like this can quickly lead to a feeling of overload.

When it comes to attention, we distinguish two important aspects. First, "alertness," or attentiveness, and second, "sustained attention." Sustained attention means the degree to which you can continue to focus on something. This, too, is a basic cognitive function: if you fail to pay close attention and keep your attention, it is very difficult to learn something new.

Third, working memory: the ability to keep information available for a short period of time so that you can edit it. An example of this is remembering a phone number so that you can dial the number shortly after someone tells you.

Declarative memory is about remembering specific information, such as a specific story. The non-declarative memory is about learning procedures, such as cycling or playing football. No abnormalities were found in the non-declarative memory in people with schizophrenia.

Finally, executive functions revolve around planning, organizing, controlling and adjusting behavior. This also includes taking initiative and starting up processes. Due to negative symptoms, it seems as if the "starting engine" is failing: you simply do not start an activity.

However, please note that there is a great deal of variation: some patients have a similar cognitive function to those without schizophrenia, while others differ greatly in all cognitive functions. Although there are clear differences at the group level between people with schizophrenia and people without schizophrenia, you cannot distinguish individuals with a disorder in the schizophrenia spectrum on the basis of cognitive function. Therefore, it is not a criterion for classification (Hanssen, Aleman and Krabbedam 2018).

How large are the abnormalities in cognitive functions in people with schizophrenia spectrum disorders?

As a group, both patients who use antipsychotics and patients who have never used antipsychotics have a slower information processing speed, less attention, a reduced memory function and more limited executive functions. The magnitude of those mean differences between people with schizophrenia and people without schizophrenia is about one standard deviation. In about 70 percent of people with schizophrenia, there are abnormalities in cognitive function (Hanssen, Aleman and Krabbedam 2018).

Figure 13.1 Distribution of cognitive function in people with or without schizophrenia

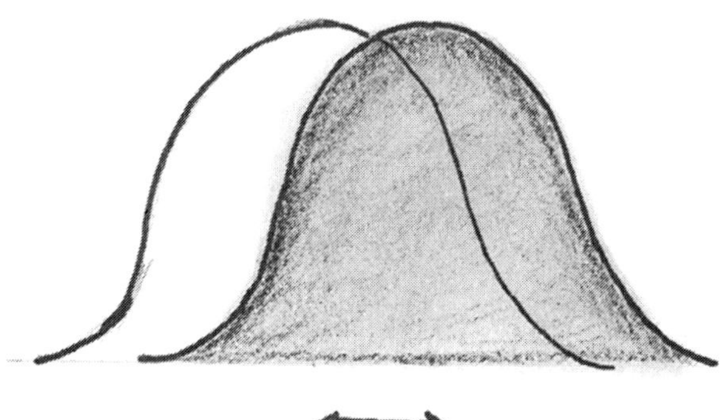

people with schizophrenia people without schizophrenia

How does cognitive impairment affect daily functioning?

Cognitive impairment is an important predictor of problems in daily functioning in patients classified with schizophrenia. Although cognitive function is one of the most important predictors, a review of the study shows that "only" 15 percent of the variation in daily functioning is explained by cognitive dysfunction. In other words, even with an important predictor, there are many other factors that largely determine the outcome (Hanssen, Aleman and Krabbedam 2018).

What is the effect of antipsychotics on cognitive function?

Research shows that antipsychotics in general have a small beneficial effect on cognitive functioning. Newer antipsychotics, such as olanzapine or quetiapine, possibly showed a slightly larger effect than other antipsychotics (the effect size is approximately 0.20 or less). This could be because these agents block the dopamine receptor somewhat less robustly, while at therapeutic doses they do not clearly lead to drowsiness. However, it could also be because the older antipsychotics were dosed too high. In other words, the comparison was not entirely fair in the studies conducted. After all, a dose that is too high slows down too much, therefore causing troubles with attention. It is therefore uncertain whether there is a real difference in the influence on cognitive function between antipsychotics.

What is the course of neurocognitive problems?

Neurocognitive impairment may occur because patients perform worse when they are distracted by voices or delusions. But that certainly does not explain everything. In people who later meet the criteria for a schizophrenia spectrum disorder, cognitive function disorders (in attention, memory and verbal reasoning) are present on average during childhood. This has been well researched in groups. On average, these functional problems increase immediately before the psychosis and problems remain more or less stable afterwards. So, there is no further deterioration. Note that this concerns the average course in groups. It does not apply to all patients with a schizophrenia spectrum disorder. In the GROUP study, patients, siblings and controls, all showed an improvement in cognitive function over the course of three to six years. This course is more in line with a theory that assumes that cognitive impairments occur as a result of a developmental disorder than with a theory that assumes deterioration as a cause (Hanssen, Aleman and Krabbedam 2018).

Is there a relationship between cognitive dysfunction and other symptoms?

Neurocognitive dysfunction is associated with the severity of negative symptoms. And, unsurprisingly, reduced executive function is associated with the severity of disorganization.

Are there also neurocognitive impairments in first-degree relatives of people with schizophrenia?

Research in healthy first-degree relatives of patients shows, on average, comparable but less pronounced cognitive impairments compared to healthy control subjects than found in patients (effect size between 0.2 and 0.6).

Social cognition

Why has there been more interest in social cognition in schizophrenia research lately?

In recent years, there has been more interest in social cognition in schizophrenia research. This is primarily because many psychotic symptoms have a social aspect. An example is a paranoid delusion. Secondly, because people with schizophrenia often experience problems in social contact. A meta-analysis has shown that social cognition is indeed related to functioning in daily life. In addition, social cognition disorders were found to be a better predictor of problems in daily functioning than neurocognition (about 23 percent of the variation in daily functioning was determined by social cognition) (Hanssen, Aleman and Krabbedam 201

Which social cognitive functions are distinguished?

The following social cognitive functions have been studied in people with schizophrenia:

1 emotion perception;
2 social perception;
3 mentalizing; and
4 attribution style.

What is emotion perception?

Emotion perception is the ability to recognize and process emotional information. It is about the recognition of facial expressions and the noticing of emotion in speech. People with schizophrenia especially have trouble correctly perceiving negative emotions, such as fear and anger. In the sense that they think they see more self-centered anger in others than is real, which was found to be related to their own suspicion and fear. Emotion perception is related to social behavior and social skills. Although this association was not found in all studies.

What is social perception?

Social perception is the ability to correctly interpret social cues, both verbal and non-verbal, within a given social situation. Social perception is closely related to social knowledge. Social cues and knowledge are also highly dependent on culture. On average, people with schizophrenia have more difficulty interpreting verbal and non-verbal social cues. They make less use of context to understand social situations. Performance on social perception tasks is related to social behavior and social skills. There has also been research in which taking context into account was detrimental to performance. Patients with schizophrenia were found to perform better in those tasks. In these tasks they were not bothered by the disruptive influence of the context (Hanssen, Aleman and Krabbedam 2018).

What is mentalization?

Mentalization is the ability to assess the intentions, beliefs and state of mind of other people. A term pointing to mentalizing is "Theory of Mind". This means that you understand that the other person has their own judgment about a certain situation, and that someone else also has their own needs and ambitions. In short, you understand that someone else has their own way of processing information and that someone can think and perceive differently than you. On average, people with schizophrenia perform well over one standard deviation lower on Theory of Mind tasks than people without schizophrenia. This appears to be an important predictor of functioning in daily life. In a study of a game situation, patients with schizophrenia had less confidence in their opponent. You can imagine that social problems increase if you don't trust others. Similar problems can occur with people with autism (Hanssen, Aleman and Krabbedam 2018).

What is attribution style?

Attribution style is the way people generally think about explanations for certain events. A distinction is made between internal and external attributions. With internal attributions, someone puts the cause on himself. With external attributions, someone places the cause of an event on factors outside of himself. A number of studies have shown that patients with a schizophrenia spectrum disorder are more likely to place the cause of negative events outside of themselves and rather to another person than to a particular situation. But a number of other studies did not find this difference.

What are the consequences of reduced social understanding?

Delusions, less social contact and social cognitive disorders can cause people with schizophrenia to have negative thoughts about others. That could also be the reason that sometimes intimate relationships don't work out well.

What is the course of social cognitive dysfunction?

Research during the phase before, during and after the first psychosis found comparable social-cognitive function disorders in patients. These problems are therefore likely to have a stable character and are not related to the varying severity of psychotic symptoms.

Are social-cognitive problems also found in family members of patients?

Family members of patients with schizophrenia perform slightly less well on average on Theory of Mind tasks and on social cognitive tasks, and they trust opponents slightly less in a test setup. However, they increase their trust in others more easily when they receive reassuring information about an opponent than patients with schizophrenia. Perhaps the fact that relatives are easier to reassure is related to the fact that they do not suffer from psychotic symptoms (Hanssen, Aleman and Krabbedam 2018).

Metacognition

Which metacognitive functions have been studied in schizophrenia?

The following metacognitive aspects have been investigated:

1 illness insight;
2 hastily drawing conclusions; and
3 monitoring self-generated actions.

What deviations in the understanding of disease occur in patients with schizophrenia?

Many patients with a psychotic illness feel that they are all right and that they do not need treatment. This actually makes a lot of sense. When you are completely convinced of something, you cannot put it into perspective or look at it from another angle. Insight into psychosis is mostly not a matter of all or nothing: patients can have insight into psychosis to a greater or lesser extent. Some realize they have a psychiatric illness, others recognize psychotic symptoms as abnormal experiences, and still others see the need for treatment. The relationship between what patients think is not always completely logical. For example, some people do not think they have any disease at all, but they find drug treatment very acceptable. Or they think they are ill because they are taking medication.

What are the causes of less "insight into psychosis"?

In the first place, less insight could be related to the fundamental problem that psychotic experiences and beliefs are so impressive and important that they cannot be put into perspective. Perhaps it also has to do with reduced self-evaluation or self-reflection.

Do patients with schizophrenia tend to jump to conclusions?

This question was investigated with the so-called bead task. People are asked to judge from which vase a bead comes. One vase has 80 percent red and 20 percent blue beads and the other vase has 20 percent red and 80 percent blue beads. The subject does not get to see the vases, but one bead is removed and shown to him or her. The test subject can then decide that he knows enough from which vase the bead comes or ask for another bead from the same vase. Patients can already decide which vase the beads come from on the basis of few beads. They make decisions based on little evidence and are also more confident in their decisions. This tendency is called "jumping to conclusions". On average, this tendency was mainly found in patients who suffered from delusions (Hanssen, Aleman and Krabbedam 2018).

What is meant by Self-Generated Actions Monitoring?

Monitoring of self-generated actions is also referred to as self-monitoring. It is the ability to estimate whether actions are caused by you or not. Examples of "actions" are speaking, moving and talking to yourself (also called internal speech). In internal speech you talk in your head. You give words to your stream of thoughts. In the brain, a distinction is made between stimuli that come from outside and sensations that are produced by someone themselves, and therefore come from within. Self-monitoring is the mechanism that assesses whether actions come from within or from outside. The brain continuously predicts the sensory consequences (consequences for sensory perception) of actions generated by the person. An example: when you lift a box, your body already estimates how it will feel, how heavy it will be. If the box turns out to be much lighter or heavier than you thought, the sensory predictions will not come true, and that stands out. At the time of that "prediction error", dopamine is also highly active (see also Chapter 16 on basic sense of self and chapter 19 on dopamine). You notice it.

Do patients have trouble monitoring self-generated actions?

A meta-analysis showed that people with schizophrenia who suffered from hallucinations have more difficulty assessing whether information comes from outside or inside.

The prediction mechanism is slightly less accurate in people with schizophrenia. As a result, the consequences of an action generated by patients themselves stand out. The consequences felt more surprising, they were not expected. This gives the impression that the origin of the experience is outside the person.

Which cognitive dysfunction can be associated with hallucinations?

In the first place, difficulty with self-monitoring can, as stated above, make it difficult for patients to determine whether experiences come from outside or from within. In addition, patients may be more likely to detect something meaningful in unstructured information.

Which cognitive impairments can be associated with delusions?

The tendency to draw conclusions on the basis of little information is related to the development and persistence of delusions. In addition, there is also a tendency to think that other persons are the cause of events related to it. Some patients with paranoid delusions tend to attribute too many (negative) intentions to other people. With delusions they try to explain why they perceive something that initially seemed strange and very important. Once they have a delusional belief, what was previously so striking and strange becomes easier to understand (for further discussion of this see also Chapter 19 on dopamine)

References

Hanssen Esther, Aleman Andre, Krabbedam Lydia. 2018. "Cognitieve stoornissen" In Handboek schizofreniespectrumstoornissen, edited by Wiepke Cahn, Inez Myin-Germeys, Richard Bruggeman, Lieuwe de Haan. Amsterdam: De Tijdstroom.

PART 5.

RISK FACTORS AND UNDERLYING MECHANISMS

The questions and answers described in this section are often complex. It can be difficult to understand the information, especially if you didn't study biology in high school. This is especially true of the chapters on genes, biological risk factors, the brain and the immune system. If you decide not to read these chapters, you will not miss information that is important for understanding the symptoms of psychosis and schizophrenia or the treatment. If you want to understand what research into the biology of psychosis and schizophrenia is about, you can read these chapters.

Chapter 16 on basic sense of self self and chapter 19 on dopamine, on the other hand, are important for understanding the development of psychotic symptoms. These chapters are more comprehensive than the others, more important to read and also provide more examples.

CHAPTER 14

GENES

What is a gene?

A gene is part of the DNA that contains the code for the production of a particular protein. You could see a gene as the blueprint for a protein. It is estimated that humans have about 20.000 genes.

Genes are located on chromosomes. Chromosomes consist of coiled DNA. Each human cell contains about 2 meters of DNA! Humans have 23 pairs of chromosomes. You also have a copy of each chromosome, so 46 chromosomes in total. Sometimes during fertilization, the copying and reassembling of chromosomes goes wrong. For example in Down's syndrome, where chromosome 21 is present in three copies instead of a duplicate.

What is DNA?

DNA is the abbreviation for Deoxyribo Nucleic Acid. DNA is a complex molecule (literally!) Made up of two long strands of nucleotides. Nucleotides are the building blocks of DNA. The two strands are connected in a double spiral shape. There are only four types of nucleotides, which are indicated with the letters A, T, G and C. They always form the same connections with each other: A can only bind with T and G only with C. Both DNA strands fit therefore exactly on top of each other. The strands can separate and then make exactly the same combination again with two new strands. Then you have two identical DNA spirals. Just as you can make words and sentences with letters, the letters of the DNA are also used to code hereditary information. We do not yet know exactly the function of large parts of the DNA.

How is the genetic code translated into proteins?

As mentioned, a gene is part of the DNA that contains the code for the production of a certain protein. Proteins are the building blocks of the organism and of biological processes. They are made up of so-called amino acids. Three letters of the DNA (for example nucleotides C, A, and T) form the code for one of the twenty existing amino acids. The sequence of letters in the DNA determines the sequence of amino acids in the protein, and thus its function. You can compare different amino acids with different colored and shaped Lego blocks. Several of these Lego blocks in a certain order together form a protein structure. Protein structures, in turn, are also building blocks. You can build cells with proteins, but you can also make hormones or enzymes.

An important part of the DNA is not involved in the coding of proteins, nor in regulating the activity of a gene. As indicated earlier, we do not yet know exactly the function of large parts of the DNA.

All the genetic information of an organism together is called the genome.

Figure 14.1 Cell, chromosome, gene

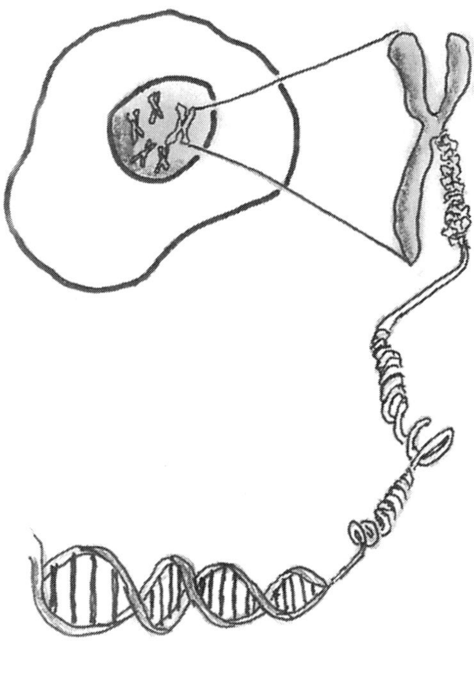

Figure 14.2 DNA

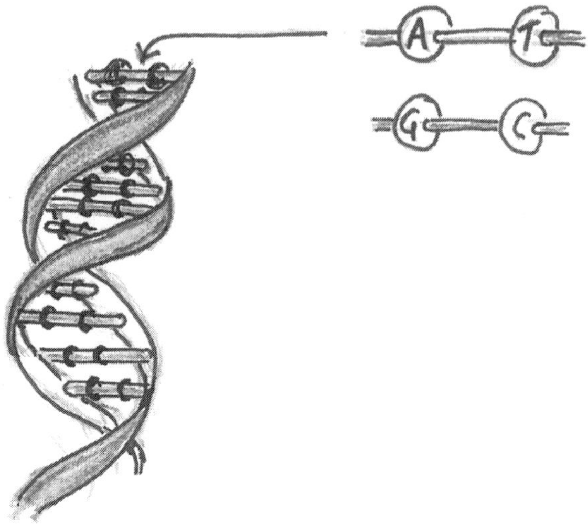

How have twin studies contributed to our knowledge of heredity in schizophrenia?

If twins both meet the classification schizophrenia, this is called concordance. The degree of concordance can be examined in a group of identical twins (which are nearly 100 percent genetically identical) and a group of fraternal twins (which are about 50 percent genetically identical). The schizophrenia twin studies show that the concordance is about 50 percent in monozygotic twins and between 4 and 15 percent in fraternal twins. This shows that if you have more of the same genes, you are more likely to have the same condition. But this also shows that genes are not the only factor that determines whether someone develops schizophrenia. If so, the concordance in identical twins would be 100 percent.

And then you could also argue that identical twins have more of the same upbringing and also experience the same circumstances in their lives. In other words, factors other than genes could be the cause of the concordance. That is why it was examined whether the situation during childhood has a major influence on the concordance. That turns out not to be the case. In monozygotic twins adopted in different families, the concordance was about the same as in monozygotic twins growing up in the same family.

What is the estimated heritability of schizophrenia (and what does this mean)?

The estimated heritability of schizophrenia is about 80 percent. This means that 80 percent of the variation in vulnerability to schizophrenia in the population can be explained by variation in genes. That is a very high percentage. However, this percentage also includes the contribution of environmental influences associated with variation in genes: gene-environment interaction and gene-environment correlation. In short, these terms boil down to the fact that some genes only cause problems with a certain environmental factor (gene-environment interaction) or that some genes increase the chance of experiencing some influences from the environment (gene-environment correlation). These concepts are explained later in this chapter, but the story boils down to fact that a high percentage of heredity also includes an important contribution from environmental factors.

This 80 percent estimated heritability also does not mean that there is an 80 percent chance that a child will meet the classification schizophrenia if the disease runs in a family. The genetic vulnerability to schizophrenia and schizophrenia spectrum disorders is caused by very many small genetic differences. Everyone carries a fair amount of these risk genes. It is believed that only when the amount of vulnerability genes exceeds a certain threshold does a greater vulnerability develop. Again, the high heritability estimate certainly does not mean that environmental risk factors play only a minor role. The high heritability does mean that a large part of the vulnerability arises in the interaction between what someone experiences (these are the risk factors from the environment) and genetic vulnerability.

What is the risk of recurrence of schizophrenia if schizophrenia occurs within a family?

"The recurrence risk" of schizophrenia is the probability that someone will meet the classification schizophrenia if someone else in the family meets this classification. The recurrence risk depends on the genetic relationship you have with a family member with schizophrenia:

If someone has an identical twin sister or brother with schizophrenia, then the chance is 50 percent that he or she will also develop schizophrenia.

If a first-degree family member (father, mother, or brother or sister) has schizophrenia, the risk that another sibling will also meet the schizophrenia classification is about 9 percent.

If a second-degree family member (e.g. grandfather, grandmother, uncle, aunt) has schizophrenia, the risk of a child later meeting the schizophrenia classification is about 3 percent.

If a third-degree family member has schizophrenia, the risk that a child will meet the schizophrenia classification is approximately 1.5 percent.

If schizophrenia does not run in the family, the risk that someone will one day meet the classification schizophrenia is about 0.5 percent.

What different forms of genetic research are there?

Linkage research examines whether a particular region of DNA is more common in family members who meet the classification of schizophrenia. If so, "that DNA region" travels with the disease, and the area around that marked spot is more likely to be related to vulnerability to the disease.

In association research it is investigated whether variation in a certain nucleotide at a certain place in the DNA is related to the classification of schizophrenia. Association research is thus more detailed than linkage research. Association research involves one different "letter" in the genetic code. Large groups of patients are compared with large groups of people without the classification schizophrenia. You can do this research if you already have an idea in advance about the possible involvement of a particular gene. You can also look for differences between people with and without schizophrenia without having a theory beforehand. If you investigate this over the entire genome (ie all the genetic information of the organism), you speak of a "*genome wide association study*" (GWAS). Because the influence of individual genes on the risk of developing schizophrenia is very small and because you have to be careful not to make many random findings because you are examining so many genes at the same time, you need very large groups of people. You have to take into account finding coincidental associations, because you are investigating so many associations at the same time. That is why you have to set very strict requirements for the level of significance. Only when the chance that you make an accidental finding is less than about 0.000001 percent, is the finding relevant. More than 10,000 people are therefore needed for this type of research.

With a *Polygenic Risk Score*, you add up all those genes that only slightly increase the risk. The very small influence of all nucleotides that were found to be abnormal is added together to a composite risk score. Incidentally, instead of just looking at risk, you can of course also check whether certain genetic characteristics make someone more resilient. This research has recently started. Similarly, a Polygenic Resilience Score has been developed. The higher that score, the higher your resilience and resistance to resist a certain condition, and therefore not to get it.

You can also research the *structure of the chromosome*. Copying errors may occur in the distribution of hereditary material from your parents. That is why this is called *Copy Number Variation* (CNV). It may be that part of the chromosome is forgotten when copying. Or a part is duplicated, or reversed on the chromosome or on another chromosome. These copy errors are much less common than deviations in nucleotides at a particular location. But because it concerns so much genetic information at the same time, these copy errors often have a major impact.

Figure 14.3 Copy Number Variation

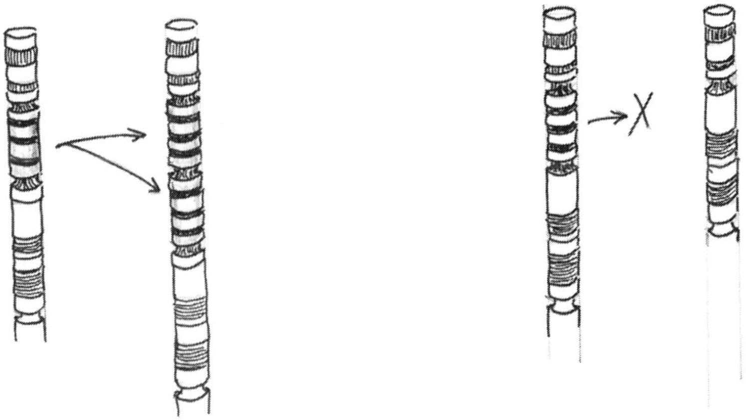

Finally, there is a new, highly detailed technique: *sequencing*. This determines the precise sequence of all nucleotides. This can also be done for the entire genome. More findings from this technique are expected in the future.

Figure 14.4 Sequencing

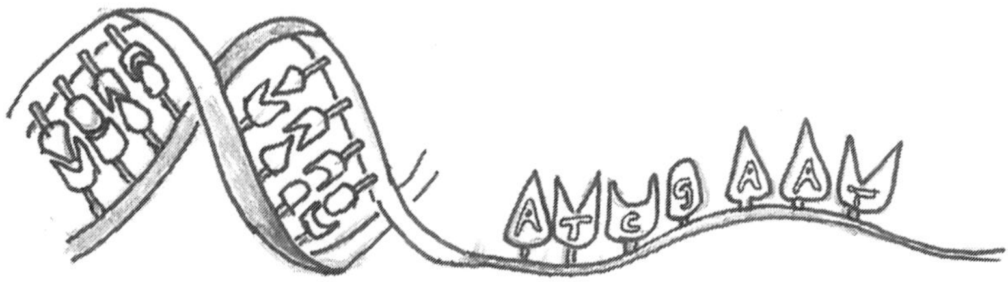

What has been found in the largest GWAS study to date?

A major GWAS study in nearly 37,000 people with schizophrenia and more than 113,000 controls found 108 areas associated with schizophrenia vulnerability. You can show this in a figure, where the likelihood of all places on the genome that they contribute to the vulnerability to schizophrenia is indicated. These types of graphs are also referred to as "Manhattan plots" because they look like the Manhattan skyline in New York. Scientists are so excited about this finding that there are even T-shirts with the Manhattan plot of this research printed on it. These findings are not yet important for the individual patient. The effect of the separate genetic variation is far too small for that. Nevertheless, this research is important because it shows abnormalities in genes involved in dopamine, glutamate, synapses and the immune system. This provides inspiration for further research into these processes. (Dopamine, glutamate, synapses, and the immune system are explained later in this section in the various chapters.) (Schizophrenia Working Group of the Psychiatric Genomics Consortium 2014)

What has been found in research with the polygenetic risk score?

The polygenetic risk score for schizophrenia was also found to be elevated in patients with bipolar disorder. This shows that the classifications schizophrenia and bipolar disorder therefore partly have the same genetic background (Purcell et al. 2009).

Another study showed a slightly greater decline in cognitive abilities with aging in healthy subjects with a high polygenetic risk score for schizophrenia. What that says exactly is not entirely clear. Perhaps some of the genes involved in the risk of schizophrenia are less beneficial in keeping certain connections or synapses in the brain vital (McIntosh et al. 2013). It was also found that a high polygenetic risk score in adolescents with schizophrenia was associated with negative symptoms and not with psychotic symptoms such as delusions and hallucinations. It may be that negative symptoms are mainly related to the genetic risk of schizophrenia (Purcell et al. 2009).

What has been found with research into Copy Number Variation (CNV)?

A CNV occurs in about 15 percent of people who meet the classification schizophrenia and in about 5 percent in the healthy population. The CNVs can be very different, and an individual CNV can have a lot of impact on a patient, but nevertheless hardly explain anything at the group level. This is because a CNV is relatively rare and therefore does not contribute much to the average of the group of patients. Perhaps the occurrence of CNV in some patients partly explains the large differences between patients.

What has been found with sequencing research?

Initial findings from sequencing research indicate the role of the NMDA receptor and calcium channels in vulnerability to schizophrenia. NMDA receptors play a role in the action of glutamate. Calcium channels are involved in the electrical currents that play a role in information transfer between nerve cells. These concepts are further explained in the chapters on dopamine and glutamate, Chapter 19 and Chapter 20 respectively.

Why is genetic research into schizophrenia so difficult?

Genetic research into schizophrenia is difficult, because patients differ not only in symptoms, but also in underlying genetic traits. Furthermore, research is difficult for two more reasons. First, because the common variation in genes found so far explains only a very small part of the risk. Second, because coarser genetic abnormalities that explain a greater proportion of the risk are rare. We still cannot explain most of the heredity. This is also because, in addition to "deviations in the construction drawing of proteins", much more can be going on in the processes that take place after "reading the construction drawing". For example, the influence of genetic variation depends on what someone experiences (gene-environment interaction). Finally, the influence of genetic variation also depends on the degree to which genes are activated or inhibited (you call this epigenetics, see below). All this together creates a dizzyingly complex puzzle. The difference between people is not only in the "construction drawing", but also in what they experience in relation to how they are "built", and in all things that can go differently during the continuous construction. You can compare it with promblems in buiding a house: "Subcontractors who do something else. Building materials that are less widely available. Pieces of the building plan that receive a lot of attention while other parts are being scaled down."

What is meant by gene-environment interaction?

Gene-environment interaction means that the effect of a certain genetic variation mainly occurs when someone experiences certain things. For example, you will only notice a difference in certain genetic variation when people start using cannabis. Only if you have a certain genetic variant, the risk of psychosis from cannabis use is greatly increased. There is then an interaction between a certain genetic sensitivity and a certain environmental factor. This interaction can of course also be positive. Some people are better able to cope with the disruptive effects of some environmental influence than others. You also call this gene-environment interaction.

What is meant by gene-environment correlation?

In gen-environment correlation, the degree of exposure to certain environmental influences depends on genetic variation. For example, you can imagine that someone who is less anxious and more impulsive due to genetic variation starts taking drug use more easily. In other words, a certain genetic trait makes it more likely that someone will experience something. Gene and environment then occur together. Then they are correlated.

What are the findings of gene-environment interaction studies in schizophrenia?

This research can be divided into two types: the omnibus approach and candidate gene research.

In the omnibus approach, you examine groups that differ in genetic vulnerability. You don't look at the genetic code, but you compare groups that differ in genetic susceptibility to schizophrenia. For example, siblings of patients with schizophrenia and people without a family member with schizophrenia. Then you check whether the genetically vulnerable group reacts differently to a risk factor from the environment. In this way it has been shown that people with a (slightly) increased genetic vulnerability (such as brothers and sisters) suffer more from mild psychotic symptoms when they use cannabis than people without genetic vulnerability.

Candidate gene research examines whether a certain genetic variation (which has been chosen because we believe that a certain genetic variation is important in the biology of vulnerability) interacts with a certain risk factor from the environment. This has been done with a variation of the gene that codes for the enzyme COMT, which breaks down dopamine. There are several variants of that enzyme. Some varieties break down dopamine quickly and others do it slowly. The first study found that people who had a variation of the COMT gene were ten times more likely to develop schizophrenia spectrum disorder when using cannabis than people without this variant. Before accepting such a finding, it is important that other researchers find the same thing when they repeat the study on another group of people. Some studies confirmed the original finding, but the studies that repeated the original study very precisely did not find this association. In short, whether this finding is really true is uncertain. However, several studies have found that interaction between the genes that code for another enzyme (AKT1) and cannabis use increases the risk of a psychotic disorder (Vorstman and Kahn 2018).

Why is gene-environment interaction research with candidate gene research so difficult?

Gene-environment interaction research with candidate gene research is complex, because we're looking for a needle in a haystack. 99.9 percent of humans have the same genome. Genetic differences are in 0.1 percent of the genome. But in that 0.1 percent, differences can occur in 10 to 15 million places. A place on the genome where there is a difference between individuals is called a polymorphism. Now it is very difficult to choose the "right" polymorphism to investigate. We still know too little about the precise function of proteins for which the genes code. Moreover, those genes and proteins do not operate on their own. They influence each other, which makes it even more complex. In addition, you have to take into account the chance that you will find something by chance. The risk of a chance finding increases when you investigate many interactions. If you examine a hundred connections between the cases, a number of connections will be found by chance alone, when these connections are actually irrelevant.

Furthermore, there is a problem that plays a role in all research: positive findings (if you find a connection) are published much more easily than negative findings (you cannot find a connection). Researchers are just humans: if you don't find something, it's not fun and boring and so there is a good chance that negative findings will not be published. But this gives us an incorrect image of reality. You call this a "bias". A bias indicates a distortion of reality. This type of bias is called publication bias.

A solution for the gene environment research could be to investigate the interaction between genetic variation and environmental factors in very large groups of people, such as in the above-mentioned GWAS studies. The problem here, however, is that you have to measure the environmental factors precisely and reliably for all those ten to one hundred thousand people. That is very difficult. Collecting blood and determining the genetic code is possible on a large scale in a standardized way. But capturing environmental factors very precisely and reliably is a huge job in such a large group (Vorstman and Kahn 2018).

What is Epigenetics?

Epigenetics studies the part of the hereditary regulation of genes that is not recorded in the DNA code. The degree to which a particular gene is active - this is also called gene expression - and how much protein is made depends on many factors. In other words, it is not only about what the "construction drawing" looks like, but also about whether and how often the construction drawing is read and converted into a part of the actual building. Environmental factors such as stress and the use of medication or smoking can also influence gene expression (Vorstman and Kahn 2018).

Is there reason to conduct genetic research in health care on patients with certain characteristics?

The risk of a CNV is higher in patients who have certain additional problems. Sometimes it can be wise to find out through genetic research, because then you can take into account problems that may be related to these hereditary characteristics. These may be patients with certain congenital abnormalities, such as a defective heart valve or epilepsy, or patients with a clear developmental disorder or an intellectual disability (Vorstman and Kahn 2018).

What is pharmacogenetics and what are the benefits?

Pharmacogenetics investigates the influence of genes on the response to drugs. There are certain genetic variants that affect the effectiveness of enzymes that remove antipsychotics from the body. For example, if you have a gene that makes your enzymes work more slowly, then there is a good chance that with an average dose of a medicine you will get a much too high blood level. In addition, genetic variation is also associated with certain side effects of medications, such as the risk of tardive dyskinesia, a movement disorder, or the risk of a reduction in white blood cells during treatment with clozapine. We will discuss this in Chapter 41 on antipsychotics (Vorstman and Kahn 2018).

Why does schizophrenia persist in the future?

People who have suffered from schizophrenia spectrum disorder are less likely to have children than people who do not. Because the contribution of hereditary vulnerability is so high, you would expect that the number of people with schizophrenia would decrease over time. That does not happen. Most studies show that the incidence (the percentage of people who meet the classification schizophrenia for the first time in a given period) of schizophrenia remains constant. An explanation for this could be that the genes that increase vulnerability also have beneficial properties at the same time. It may be that the genes that increase the sensitivity of the dopamine system are also associated with "being entrepreneurial", "being creative or original". Those are qualities that actually help in finding a partner and having offspring. So, the vulnerability to schizophrenia could remain constant in the population, because it is related to the beneficial characteristics of people. There is also scientific support for this idea: certain genetic variation is associated with poorer cognitive function in patients with schizophrenia, but the same genetic variation is associated with better cognitive function in family members and in healthy participants.

In short, what good is genetics?

Genetics is not going to provide simple answers to complex questions. It turns out to be much more complex than we thought 25 years ago. It has become clear that we need to investigate very large groups of people to gain reliable and valuable knowledge of the genetic variation associated with vulnerability. Moreover, it has become clear that genetic vulnerability does not adhere to the classifications we have devised. In fact, everyone carries dozens to hundreds of genes that increase vulnerability to psychosis.

But what good is genetic research? In the short term, for the readers of this book, little or nothing, indeed. Perhaps a lot in the long run. In the first place, it helps us unravel the complex biological pathway of vulnerability. In the second place, it could help us in the future to distinguish different routes to vulnerability to schizophrenia, for example: for one patient mainly via a dysregulation of the immune system and for the other mainly through a dysregulation of the feedback mechanisms of the dopamine system. Knowing more about this could help us look for treatments that not only suppress symptoms, but address the cause of the dysregulation (Vorstman and Kahn 2018).

References

McIntosh, A.M., Gow, A., Luciano, M., Davies, G., Liewald, D.C., Harris, S.E., e.a. (2013). Polygenic risk for schizophrenia is associated with cognitive change between childhood and old age. *Biological Psychiatry, 73,* 938-943.

Purcell, S.M., Wray, N.R., Stone, J.L., Visscher, P.M., O'Donovan, M.C., Sullivan PF, e.a. (2009). Common polygenic variation contributes to risk of schizophrenia and bipolar disorder. *Nature,*

Schizophrenia Working Group of the Psychiatric Genomics Consortium (2014). Biological insights from 108 schizophrenia-associated genetic loci. *Nature, 511,* 421-427.

Vorstman, Jacob, Kahn, Rene. 2018. "Genetica" In Handboek schizofreniespectrumstoornissen, edited by Wiepke Cahn, Inez Myin-Germeys, Richard Bruggeman, Lieuwe de Haan. Amsterdam: De Tijdstroom.

CHAPTER 15

PSYCHOSOCIAL RISK FACTORS

In earlier days some theorists used to think that a cold relationship with "double binding" with the mother could cause schizophrenia. Double binding mend that you were always a failure. A worthless and horrible idea that was based on nothing and has deeply hurt many mothers! Others saw the diagnosis of schizophrenia as society's way of getting rid of troublesome individuals. In other cultures, schizophrenia is sometimes seen as a punishment from God or a spell.

These erroneous and embarrassing theories have left research on psychosocial risk factors underexposed for a while. With such a history, people did not dare to investigate social factors that increased the risk of schizophrenia spectrum disorders. However, this hesitation has disappeared in the last fifteen years.

What are Psychosocial Risk Factors?

Psychosocial risk factors are conditions or events in the social environment that affect a person's psychological characteristics, vulnerability or condition.

In the following I will answer questions concerning the following social factors:

1 growing up in a big city;
2 migration;
3 childhood trauma;
4 life events.

Growing up in a big city

Is the risk of psychosis increased if you grow up in a big city?

A number of meta-analyzes show that the risk of developing schizophrenia spectrum disorder is more than twice as high when you grow up in a big city than when you grow up in the countryside. The risk is especially increased if children live in the city between the ages of four and twelve. This is the age when they go out on the streets and are still developing.

Is growing up in the big city really a causal factor?

You may wonder whether the growing up in the city really causes an increased risk. It could also be that people with psychosis in the city are more in need of care than people in the countryside. Then it could be that there are just as many people with psychosis in the countryside as in the city. Research shows that this cannot explain the difference, however, because people in the city and in the countryside use mental health care equally often. It could also be that people with an increased risk of psychosis move to the city more often. You call that the selection hypothesis. But this cannot be the explanation either, because young children who moved from city to country or vice versa were exposed to the risk associated with their new place of residence. In addition, the link has been repeatedly found in different countries. And there was also a dose-response relationship: the higher the population density, the greater the risk of psychosis. In addition, exposure to the risk factor precedes psychosis. As mentioned, the risk is especially increased if children live in the city between the ages of four and twelve, while psychoses usually develop between the ages of twenty and twenty-five. In short, there are many indications that growing up in large cities is really a causal risk factor.

Which factors in the big city increase the risk?

Metropolitan stress is mentioned as the most important factor. This may include pollution, noise or social stress. Some support for the notion that social stress plays an important role comes from research that showed that people with psychosis who walk down a very busy street are more prone to overstimulation, suspicion, hallucinations and anxiety, as well as negative ideas about themselves and others.

Evidence has also been found that the risk is higher in poorer and less safe neighborhoods (Myin-Germeys and Selten 2018).

Migration

Is migration a risk factor?

A meta-analysis showed that migrants have on average a 2.9 times higher risk of schizophrenia spectrum disorder than people from the native population. There were considerable differences within the migrant group:

Migrants from developing countries had a 3.3 times higher risk.
Migrants from rich countries had a 2.3 times higher risk.
Dark-skinned migrants had a 4.8 times higher risk.

These are quite large differences, which have been found repeatedly. Another meta-analysis showed that there were no differences in the relative risk between first- and second-generation migrants: the risk is thus increased for both groups.

Some believe that these numbers may be incorrect as they may be misclassified. People with a migration background would incorrectly be classified as having a schizophrenia spectrum disorder instead of, for example, the classification mood disorder. That is why a plea is made for culture-sensitive diagnostics. Nevertheless, the lack of culture-sensitive diagnostics does not seem to be a complete explanation. Although misclassification as a cause for differences in the risk between migrants and the immigrant population can certainly not be ruled out, it does not seem to totally explain the consistent findings in research with careful diagnosis in different countries (Myin-Germeys and Selten 2018).

How can the increased risk of migrants be explained?

First, we will discuss a number of possible causes that are unlikely on the basis of research. It is not because people with an increased vulnerability migrate. It is the other way around: healthy, enterprising people migrate. It does not seem to be because migrants use drugs more often. Although it cannot be entirely ruled out that cannabis use plays a role in the increased incidence among men of North African descent. It is also probably not due to a vitamin D deficiency during pregnancy (dark skinned people make vitamin D less easily), as this does not explain the increased risk of first-generation migrants. It is probably not due to a reduced immunity to a particular virus, because that does not explain the increased incidence in the second generation.

Most researchers think that the increased incidence among migrants is mainly caused by increased social stress in a situation with limited options for coping. There are the following arguments for this explanation. First, the amount of stress migrants experience was found to be related to their risk of psychosis. Second, if migrants live in a neighborhood with many people from their own ethnic group, the risk of psychosis is lower: living among people in your own group is less stressful. And because it is less stressful, you have a lower risk of psychosis (Myin-Germeys and Selten 2018).

Childhood trauma

Is childhood trauma a risk factor for developing psychosis?

A meta-analysis shows that the risk of both a psychotic disorder and of having psychotic experiences is 2.8 times higher when a person has experienced trauma during childhood. There are also indications that the risk of psychosis increases with the severity of the trauma. Especially trauma in which children are deliberately harmed, such as sexual abuse or maltreatment, increase the risk. Being bullied in childhood also increases the risk of developing psychotic symptoms later. People with mild psychotic symptoms are also more likely to report being bullied earlier. If the trauma is related to a traffic accident, for example, then the risk is hardly or not at all increased. There are also indications that stress caused by constantly having to adapt to a new environment plays a role. Of course, moving is not the same as experiencing severe trauma, but children who move often and therefore often change schools have a slightly higher risk of psychotic symptoms later in life (Myin-Germeys and Selten 2018).

Is childhood trauma related to the course of the psychotic illness?

Experiencing childhood trauma increases the likelihood of more severe symptoms, slower recovery, and longer-lasting psychotic experiences. In addition, you are more likely to also develop anxiety or manic or depressive symptoms. In people who have experienced trauma in the past, the risk of suicide is also higher. So, childhood trauma increases the likelihood that you will develop a psychiatric condition and also makes it more likely that that the course of the condition is less favorably. Every reason, therefore, to prevent trauma as much as possible.

Life events

What are life events?

Life events are situations or events that cause a significant change in your life. This could be a positive change, for example moving to a new city, getting into a relationship or starting a new job, or a negative change, such as a breakdown in a relationship, the loss of a parent or a serious accident. A life event will more or less turn your life upside down.

Do life events influence the risk of developing psychosis?

A meta-analysis shows that experiencing life events increases the risk of developing psychosis up to three times. However, there are concerns about this result. The studies summarized in the meta-analysis are mostly small, and mostly they did not correct for the possible confounding influence of childhood trauma. So, it may be that the link between life events and psychosis is largely explained by the influence of underlying childhood trauma (Myin-Germeys and Selten 2018).

How can environmental factors influence psychosis?

How environmental factors influence psychosis is a question of an underlying common mechanism that may explain why the abovementioned psychosocial risk factors increase the risk of psychosis. Below I discuss two possible explanations: sensitization and social defeat.

What is sensitization?

With sensitization you become increasingly sensitive to an event. It may mean that you continue to respond equally strongly to an increasingly mild stressful event or that you react more and more strongly to the same stressful event.

Figure 15.1 Sensitization

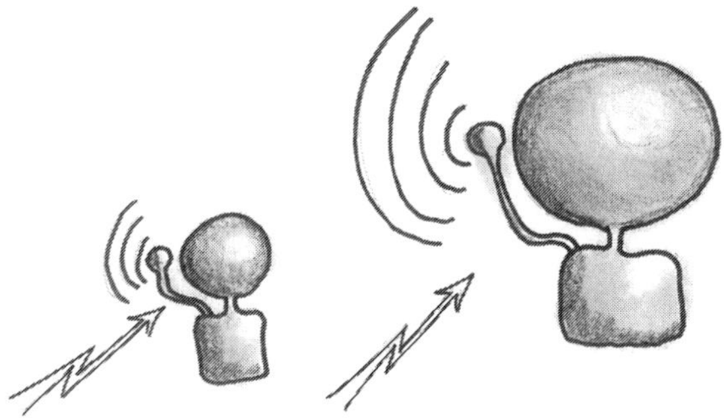

Is sensitization more common in people vulnerable to psychosis?

There are indications that sensitization is more common in people who are vulnerable to psychosis. People at risk for psychosis, people with psychosis, and also their first-degree family members react more emotionally to everyday events that are a little bit stressful (Myin-Germeys and Selten 2018).

Do trauma or life events play a role in sensitization?

It may be that the sensitivity to stress is fully genetic, but based on research findings, I believe that trauma or life events also play a role. Two studies in the general population and one study in psychotic patients showed that people who experienced trauma in childhood are more sensitive to stress. Life events in the previous year also leads to a greater emotional response to small events in daily life. From this you can deduce that your sensitivity to stress can increase if you have been through a lot of trouble (Myin-Germeys and Selten 2018).

How does sensitization increase the risk of psychosis?

It is thought that sensitization increases the risk of psychosis because a constant emotional overreaction constantly stimulates your alertness, causing you to become stressed. This increases the chance that you will develop psychotic symptoms. Stress may increase dopaminergic release.

Do trauma or discrimination damage your confidence in others, and does that subsequently contribute to the risk of psychosis?

Traumatic events or discrimination cause negative thoughts, such as the idea that you yourself are vulnerable and that others are dangerous. These negative thoughts make it easier for you to think that unpleasant events have been caused by others. You also call this external attribution. This tendency can develop further in the form of suspicious thoughts. Negative life events make you more alert to threats. As a result, you tend to interpret unclear information as threatening. Childhood trauma also affects the trust you have in others and in yourself. In addition, trauma can cause fear, sadness and loneliness. Together this can increase the risk of developing a psychotic illness. If you think that unpleasant events are caused by your own mistakes, it can also make you anxious, lonely, and depressed (Myin-Germeys and Selten 2018).

What is social defeat?

Social defeat means that someone feels defeated or humiliated by another or by a group.

What is the social defeat hypothesis of psychosis?

The social defeat hypothesis implies that prolonged humiliation or social exclusion cause increased sensitivity of the dopamine system, increasing the risk of psychosis.

Are there any research findings that support the social defeat hypothesis?

Research into the social defeat hypothesis has mainly been conducted with animals. Increased dopamine release has been found in rats that have been repeatedly beaten by another rat. The sensitivity of the dopamine system also appears to be increased. This sensitivity was greatest when the animal was isolated after defeat. The sensitivity of the dopamine system increased less when the animal returned directly to its own group after defeat. A socially familiar environment therefore reduces the impact of a bad experience. A similar sensitivity of the dopamine system has been found in patients with schizophrenia who have never used medication.

It could be that discrimination, threats, maltreatment, abuse and expulsion cause a stronger sensitivity of the dopamine system especially when people experience little support from others. This idea could explain why psychosis risk is high in people who migrated and are most likely to experience discrimination and in children who have suffered severe trauma, people who are bullied and people who are alone (Myin-Germeys and Selten 2018).

References

Myin-Germeys, Inez, Selten Jean-Paul. 2018. "Psychosociale risicofactoren" In Handboek schizofreniespectrumstoornissen, edited by Wiepke Cahn, Inez Myin-Germeys, Richard Bruggeman, Lieuwe de Haan. Amsterdam: De Tijdstroom.

CHAPTER 16

BASIC SENSE OF SELF AND PSYCHOSIS

What is a basic sense of self?

Usually, people have the feeling that they themselves perceive and that it is they themselves who think and act. When you walk down the street, look around and wonder if you will still be in time to catch the train, you feel that it is you who is walking, looking and thinking. You don't have to think about this sense of self, it comes naturally and feels common and self-evident.

What is the association between basic sense of self and psychosis?

However, if you miss this self-evident sense of self for a longer period of time, it can go hand in hand with psychosis. For example, you may have the feeling that something outside influences how you walk or think or perceive sound. Or that your movements or thoughts no longer caused by you, as you are used to. That's a strange experience.

I want to try to explain how this is possible and therefore I will describe successively: 1. how people arrive at a self-evident sense of self; 2. how you can [partially] loose a natural sense of self; 3. what the consequences may be; and 4. what you can do about it.

How do people come to have a self-evident basic sense of self?

To understand that, I first have to tell you something about how we process information, act and learn. We do that by constantly making subconscious predictions of how it will feel when something is happening. We compare these unconscious predictions with our feelings and experiences. These predictions are about what we are going to perceive, what we are going to think, what we are going to feel and about what we are going to do. These predictions are based on our past experience. You learn from birth on and you make predictions based on what you have learned. You predict something and check whether it is correct. These predictions help us to prepare for the future as best we can. Usually, our subconscious predictions are correct. If you observe, think or do something, then you experience something. If you are thirsty, look at a glass of water, think that you want to take that glass and then grab it, you will see the glass, notice that you are thinking and feel the movement of your arm and hand and the tension in your muscles, and you also feel the glass in your hand, its shape and temperature and how hard and heavy it is. If these experiences [or feelings] match your subconscious predictions exactly, then it is correct. It is going exactly as you predicted based on your past experiences. After all, you have already taken a glass many times. We continuously make predictions and constantly have experiences that match our predictions. This gives us the general feeling that "it's right". And now comes the important part. This continuous flow of "alright feelings and experiences" creates the feeling that we ourselves are the center of these feelings, perceptions, thoughts and actions. This basic sense of self thus arises from the similarity between the experiences or feelings we predict and those we actually experience. Our sensory experiences, but also our other physical feelings [muscle tension, feelings from our stomach, heartbeat and breathing] are all involved in the creation of that self-evident sense of self.

However, while most of our subconscious predictions are correct [the perceived experience matches your prediction of that experience] it is not always so. Sometimes you're wrong. You see a glass of water. You are thirsty and want to grab it. You expect it to feel cool and hard. Based on your expectations you grab the glass with a certain force, you expect to feel the hard cool glass. But if it is not glass but a transparent plastic cup with warm water, then you feel something soft and warm that you easily deform. Perhaps the plastic cup gives way under the pressure of your fingers squeezing too hard because you predicted you were going to reach for a cold hard glass. If you make a prediction error, dopamine is immediately released in your brain. Dopamine gives the signal: watch out, pay attention, something isn't right, your prediction isn't right, you have to do something else, otherwise things will go wrong. This makes you alert and full of attention. If your prediction is wrong, a dopamine signal appears, indicating that something new is happening and that you need to pay attention and act. This allows you to learn new things. This new experience allows you to adjust future predictions. As a result, your predictions in the future are better. And with all your attention you feel how to lift the plastic cup without squeezing it or sloshing the water over the edge.

Sometimes, you cannot accurately predict what will happen and what you will experience. Then you are uncertain. Then also, dopamine is released in your head. Then you pay close attention and try to reduce your uncertainty.

But most of the day your predictions are correct and you are not insecure. Because of that almost continuous stream of experiences that match your predictions, you keep the feeling that *you* observe, think and act yourself.

How can you [partially] lose a self-evident basic sense of self?

The self-evident sense of self thus arises from the convergence of virtually everything you predict with virtually everything you experience. Everything you feel, hear, see, smell and taste fits what you subconsciously predict. This is a complex and subtle process. When your predictions are not entirely correct or when different experiences do not quite fit together, the release of dopamine gives you the signal that something is going on. It is a signal that something unexpected is happening, something that is strange to you. Because it is strange and unexpected, you get the feeling that something is coming from outside, that it is not your own. If that happens repeatedly, you can lose some of your self-evident basic sense of self.

Below I discuss three examples where your predictions do not exactly match your experiences. The examples are about *walking, thinking* and *hearing voices*.

For example, you may notice that *walking* feels different than normal. Apparently, the prediction about your walking doesn't quite match what you feel in your legs and feet. Because your prediction doesn't exactly match with what you feel, dopamine is released in your head. You then start to pay more and more attention to how you walk and that makes it feel even weirder. Walking that normally comes naturally now receives a lot of conscious attention. This reduces the unconscious self-evident feeling that you are walking yourself and you may get the impression that you are not initiating or directing the walking yourself. It seems as if there is something outside that influences your walking. Because this is a disturbing feeling, you start paying more and more attention to it. Eventually you may come to believe that you are controlled by something outside of yourself. You have lost the self-evident feeling that you are walking yourself.

Something similar can also happen with *your thoughts*. Usually, your thoughts fit what you have experienced and the specific situation you are in. So, your thoughts are usually not unexpected to yourself. Apparently, there is also a kind of prediction of your thoughts subconsciously. It sometimes happens that a thought seems strange to you, so that you wonder "where did that thought come from?" But usually, the thoughts and the feelings they evoke in you fit your expectations quite well. If it often happens that thoughts do not match your prediction, you notice that. Dopamine is released in your head. You are overwhelmed by your thoughts, you repeatedly wonder where do they come from? Because you (unconsciously) did not feel them coming, the thoughts do not seem to be your own. It feels strange, disturbing, you pay even more attention to it and you can get the feeling that something outside influences your thoughts, or that the thoughts are not your own.

You can also *hear voices* when no one is talking to you nearby. This experience can arise in a similar way as described above. Thoughts and memories can come to you without you subconsciously expecting them. You really didn't see them coming. Normally, the sensitivity of your sound processing center in your head is inhibited when you subconsciously predict thoughts or memories to come. That's very useful, because you can't think or remember something and listen carefully to something else at the same time. But if you don't predict them then the sensitivity of your sound processing center is not inhibited. Thoughts or memories that you don't predict are strange to you, they don't seem to come from you. If that happens while your sound processing center is sensitive, you may experience that you actually hear those thoughts or memories and that you have the feeling that they come from outside. Because this experience does not match your prediction, it is strange to you and seems to come from outside. Because that's disturbing, even more dopamine is released in your head, which makes it even more strange and you will pay more attention to it.

Everyone makes unconscious prediction errors. In fact, by noticing unconscious prediction errors, we learn new skills and ideas. However, if too many prediction errors occur, you may be inundated with warning signs. The natural feeling that you are yourself is then under pressure. It is not exactly clear why some people suffer from prediction errors during a stressful period in their lives. Researchers think it has to do with a subtle problem in the coherent processing of feelings and experiences. In any case, it's not something that's your fault. It happens unconsciously. You can't fix it by trying harder.

What could be the consequences of a diminished basic sense of self?

You usually feel insecure when you have a less obvious sense of self. Before, it used to happen automatically, you didn't think about, now you have less grip. The world seems different and you also feel less in control. You may also lose the sense of mental privacy. Normally you know that your thoughts are private, but now it doesn't seem that way. That makes you feel vulnerable.

I described above that subtle unconscious prediction errors can give rise to impressive experiences with walking, thinking and hearing voices. These special experiences are not in accordance with your old familiar world view and beliefs about yourself. Everything seems to be different. It gives you the unsettling feeling that something must be going on, that something has changed completely. You need a new explanation for what's going on. Those experiences [for example, the feeling that you are not walking yourself, or that it is not your own thoughts that are coming into your head, or that you hear voices when no one is around to speak to you] are very impressive. Dopamine makes you alert to it and this makes you want to find out what's going on. If these experiences last longer and remain impressive, then you need a new conception of yourself and the world that can explain these experiences. There must be something special going on. This way you can get the belief that you are controlled by a force outside yourself, or that thoughts in your head come from outside, or that others speak in your head. You become convinced of this because it fits with your impressive experiences. With this new idea of yourself and the world, you better understand what you are experiencing. But you have this new belief on your own. No one else thinks that way. Others don't have your experience either. That feels lonely and that causes problems. You can get into conflicts with others because they think you shouldn't be so weird. You may feel that you are not safe anywhere and that you should therefore avoid other people. You are alone in your beliefs and you may tend to isolate yourself. This makes you think even more about your experiences and about your beliefs. Everything that you give attention grows and becomes more important. It fills your head and your experience. Others may tell you that you have delusions or hallucinations, that you have a psychosis. While you have the conviction that you and the world have changed because of those impressive experiences you have.

Another consequence of a less self-evident basic sense of self can be that you feel less motivation. You withdraw and feel less active, as if you have lost your orientation, your core motivation. The self-evident feeling that you can initiate actions seems further away.

What can you do about a diminished basic sense of self?

The subtle unconscious prediction errors that are the cause of the less self-evident sense of self cannot simply be remedied. Fortunately, there are things you can do to make it less problematic. There are at least 3 things that can help. Below I discuss them. 1. *Making dopamine less active*; 2. *Focusing attention on what you consider important in your life*; 3. *Contact with others*. These 3 actions will help reduce distressing experiences and make it more likely that you will have comforting experiences.

Decreasing dopamine activity. Dopamine becomes more active when you use drugs, when there are unconscious prediction errors, when you feel insecure or stressed, and when you have experienced something threatening.

So, the very first thing you can do is stop using drugs. Then you stop boosting dopamine and that can already help enormously.

Sometimes that's not enough to recover. Then it can help to use antipsychotics to ensure that dopamine is inhibited, so that you get fewer signals that something is not right. This makes you calmer, less alert, and you think less about everything. You can think more calmly about other things. You no longer get continuous notifications from dopamine that there are prediction errors. Because you also need dopamine for normal functioning, you should look for the lowest possible dose of antipsychotic medication that sufficiently inhibits the excessive activity of dopamine without dulling other feelings too much.

Finding an environment where you feel calm and safe and having contact with friends and family can help you feel less insecure and stressed. As a result, the activity of dopamine can decrease, so that you experience less discomfort. If your dopamine is very active, a quiet environment and contact with friends and family helps, but that alone is often not enough to recover.

If you have experienced something that was threatening, it can be traumatic. This also makes dopamine more active. You pay more attention, because you cannot be sure that you are safe. Trauma treatment can help to reduce excessive dopamine activity.

It is usually very difficult to change bad thoughts, feelings or experiences. That's also because you pay a lot of attention to bad thoughts, feelings or experiences when you try to change them. And everything that you give attention grows. That's why it can help to *focus your attention on other things that you find valuable*. That can be anything that is valuable to you: music, nature, art, sports, friends, family, learning, or work. What matters is that it is valuable to you. This will give you more reassuring and pleasant experiences. In addition, you may become less aware of strange and disturbing experiences. The net effect is that problems with your self-evident basic sense of self are less prominent and your self-confidence increases.

Connect with others. The disturbing experiences, the beliefs you got from them and reduced motivation make you tend to avoid other people. This makes you stuck in your own thoughts. As a result, you will find yourself increasingly alone. That's bad, because we humans need each other. You need contact with friends and family to feel safe, calm and connected. And contact with others may help you to focus on other things than your individual thoughts. It especially helps if you can focus on things that you both find important and can do together. Make music together, or listen to music, play sports, play games, study, work, walk and travel.

CHAPTER 17

BIOLOGICAL RISK FACTORS

What are Biological Risk Factors?

In addition to genes, there are also other biological processes or factors that can increase the vulnerability to develop a psychotic disorder. Some risk factors can be avoided. If a biological risk factor is avoided, the risk of a psychotic illness also decreases. That is, if the risk factor is really a causal factor. Below I answer questions about three types of biological risk factors: cannabis, infections and complications during pregnancy and around birth.

Cannabis

Is cannabis use a risk factor? And what is the risk?

Cannabis use is associated with a two to three times higher risk of a psychotic disorder. This figure comes from some meta-analyzes. The average risk of developing a psychotic illness at some point in your life is 4 percent. If you use cannabis, you increase that risk to 8 to 16 percent. Then you still have an 84 to 92 percent chance of not getting psychosis. That may sound reassuring, but if your risk to begin with is higher, for example because there are people in your family who have had a psychosis, then the perspective is less favorable. Suppose your initial risk is not 4 but 10 percent due to genetic sensitivity. If you then start smoking, you may increase your risk of developing a psychotic disorder to about 20 to 30 percent! And when you start early with cannabis use, say before you are 15 years, than the risk is even 4 times higher. So, the risk to develop a psychotic disorder may become as high as 40%.

Are there other factors that increase the risk of cannabis use?

The younger a person is when he starts smoking, the higher the risk. If someone starts before the age of fifteen, the risk is about four times as high that they will develop psychosis later. A large international study of first-episode psychosis found that the risk of psychosis depended strongly on the average THC content of the cannabis used in that area. The risk was exactly related to the average THC level at that location. So, the higher the THC content, the higher the risk (Diforti et al., 2018). In addition, the risk depends on a person's genetic susceptibility to psychosis. People with severe traumatic experiences in their childhood also have a higher risk of developing psychosis if they start smoking cannabis.

Is cannabis use a causal factor?

The finding that cannabis use is more common in people who develop psychotic symptoms does not necessarily mean that cannabis use is a causal factor. After all, it could also be that people with emerging psychotic symptoms use cannabis more often, for example to have fewer problems with some symptoms. This is called the self-medication hypothesis. Then the relationship would be the other way around: psychosis leads to cannabis use.

The degree to which it is likely that a particular factor is actually causal is tested on the basis of a number of criteria:

1. How large is the relationship? As mentioned above, the relationship between cannabis use and psychosis risk is robust.
2. Is the association found repeatedly? The association is found in many studies.
3. How strong is the dose-response relationship? Many studies have found a clear dose-response relationship between the degree of cannabis use and the risk of psychosis. The more often people used to smoke and the stronger the cannabis (the higher the THC content), the higher the risk of psychosis. The group of people who used to smoke the most had a four times greater risk of psychosis (Diforti et al., 2018).
4. Does the risk factor precede the condition? Initial cannabis use predicted psychotic symptoms four to seven years later. Conversely, psychotic symptoms on a first measurement did not predict cannabis use four to seven years later. However, there are studies that show that cannabis use predicts psychotic symptoms, but there are also studies that indicate that having psychotic symptoms predicts the likelihood of later cannabis use. So, there is evidence that cannabis use precedes psychosis, but vice versa, there is also evidence that psychosis sometimes precedes cannabis use.
5. Is the risk specific? The link between cannabis use and psychosis is much larger than the link between cannabis use and depression,

although the link between cannabis use and mania also seems to exist.

6. Do cannabis and psychosis co-occur due to another factor they have in common? It could be that the same genes that increase vulnerability to psychosis also increase the risk of cannabis use. This phenomenon is called gene-environment correlation (see Chapter 14 on genes). Some studies found no evidence of increased cannabis use in family members of patients with psychosis, but one study did. Two genetic studies found a small association between genetic risk of schizophrenia and cannabis use. Thus, there is some evidence that gene-environment correlation may explain a limited part of the link between cannabis use and psychosis. It could also be that other factors associated with cannabis use are causative factors for the development of psychosis. In other words, it is not the cannabis specifically that is a cause, but that other associated factors are the cause. Young people with attention problems, young people with great impulsivity and young people who grow up in less favorable socio-economic circumstances, for example, are more likely to smoke cannabis and also more often develop psychosis. However, this has been taken into account in the study of the magnitude of the association between cannabis use and psychosis. These studies have "corrected for these other factors". This means that the influence of those other factors was taken into account in the analysis. Even then, the "net" link between cannabis use and psychosis remained.
7. A biological mechanism explaining the link between cannabis and psychosis could be the increase in dopamine release. Indeed, this has been found in a number of studies.

All in all, there is considerable evidence that cannabis is a causal risk factor for developing psychosis.

How does cannabis use affect the course of psychotic illness?

Patients who smoke cannabis more often have psychotic episodes, are more often admitted to hospital, have more severe psychotic symptoms, exhibit more aggressive behavior and function less well than patients who do not smoke. Cannabis use is associated with a poorer working memory and a slower speed of information processing. Plenty of reasons to stop smoking cannabis. Still, people sometimes think they get down and even more psychotic when they stop smoking. Research and clinical experience show that this is not the case. Mood and psychosis improve when someone stops smoking cannabis.

Infections

Why are infections thought to increase the risk of schizophrenia?

Infections are thought to increase the risk of schizophrenia because variation in genes involved in the immune system is associated with schizophrenia. In addition, certain immunological conditions are more common in people with a psychotic disorder. Also, the fact that patients with schizophrenia are slightly more likely to be born at the end of winter or early spring could be associated with more infections during pregnancy. In addition, certain infections of the brain can cause psychotic symptoms. On the other hand, the largest study to date on this has found no link between maternal antibodies and the child's risk of schizophrenia. Also, in a recent meta-analysis no association was found between influenza epidemics and the risk of schizophrenia (Van Winkel, De Witte, Marcelis. 2018).

Most evidence exists for the association between infection with a particular microorganism, toxoplasma, and the risk of schizophrenia. However, this risk is not specific to schizophrenia, because bipolar disorder, obsessive-compulsive disorder or addiction problems are also seen more often after toxoplasma infection. Toxoplasma is a microorganism that can be transmitted from cats to other mammals (and humans). About 30% of the world's population has been infected with toxoplasma (Sutherland et al 2015).

A hypothesis that infections play a role, so what?

At the moment the practical consequences of this hypothesis are not substantial. At most, you could try to prevent toxoplasmosis contamination (major sources of contamination are the litter box and raw meat). Of course, if future research provides more evidence of the role of infections, it could be very important for prevention and perhaps also for the treatment of schizophrenia.

Complications in pregnancy and around birth

What are pregnancy and birth complications?

Complications during pregnancy and around birth are divided into complications during pregnancy (e.g. diabetes of the mother, malnutrition, low birth weight, birth defects, small head of the developing baby, infections, severe stress in the mother) and complications surrounding the delivery (for example birth complications such as oxygen deprivation, fluid in the lungs, emergency caesarean section and premature birth).

To what extent do pregnancy and birth complications increase the risk of schizophrenia spectrum disorders?

Various studies in which all complications surrounding pregnancy and birth have been taken together show that the risk of a schizophrenia spectrum disorder is twice as high if there is a complication in the pregnancy or around birth (Van Winkel, De Witte, Marcelis. 2018).

How can this relationship be explained?

We do not know exactly how the relationship between these complications and schizophrenia spectrum disorders can be explained. There are several ideas. Short-term oxygen deprivation during labor could cause subtle brain damage. It could also be that stress hormones that are released with many of the mentioned complications can be harmful to the brain of the developing child. Or the substances released during an increased immune response may damage the developing brain. This may include damage to the hippocampus, which causes an increased sensitivity to stress that causes more dopamine to be released during stressful situations.

Conversely, does genetic vulnerability also influence the risk of pregnancy and birth complications?

Various studies have found that especially in children with a genetically increased vulnerability, pregnancy and birth complications have a strong risk-increasing effect. This is an example of gene-environment interaction.

What is the influence of the accumulation of risk factors?

Often the various factors mentioned in this chapter occur simultaneously. Migration can, for example, be related to traumatic experiences and growing up in a big city or living in a neighborhood with a lot of stress, bullying at school and feelings of social defeat and genetic vulnerability. Research has shown that such an accumulation of risk factors has a greater effect than you would expect based on the sum of the individual risk factors.

References

Van Winkel, De Witte, Marcelis. 2018. “Biologische risicofactoren” In Handboek schizofreniespectrumstoornissen, edited by Wiepke Cahn, Inez

Myin-Germeys, Richard Bruggeman, Lieuwe de Haan. Amsterdam: De Tijdstroom.

Sutterland, A.L., Fond, G., Kuin, A., Koeter, M.W., Lutter, R., Gool, T. van, e.a. (2015). Beyond the association. Toxoplasma gondii in schizophrenia, bipolar disorder, and addiction: systematic review and meta-analysis. Acta Psychiatr Scand, 132(3), 161-179.

CHAPTER 18

BRAIN

Books have been written about the brain and its function. It is an interesting subject, but it is complex. We already know quite a bit, but there are also many uncertainties. In the following I answer questions about the brain and brain networks in broad lines. If you study the following chapter, then you know about as much as an average medical doctor.

Before you start reading, it is important to realize that the abnormalities found in people with schizophrenia are very subtle. You can never tell from a picture of the brain who has schizophrenia and who doesn't. I think that you should not see schizophrenia as a brain disease. However, a subtle disrupted development of the brain can make someone more sensitive to psychosis. Our brains are involved in everything we do and experience, so it is obvious that there may also be abnormalities in the brain associated with special experiences, delusions and negative symptoms. But that does not mean that it is all fixed. Brains change over the course of your life. What you do and experience affects your brain.

Figure 18.1 Brain

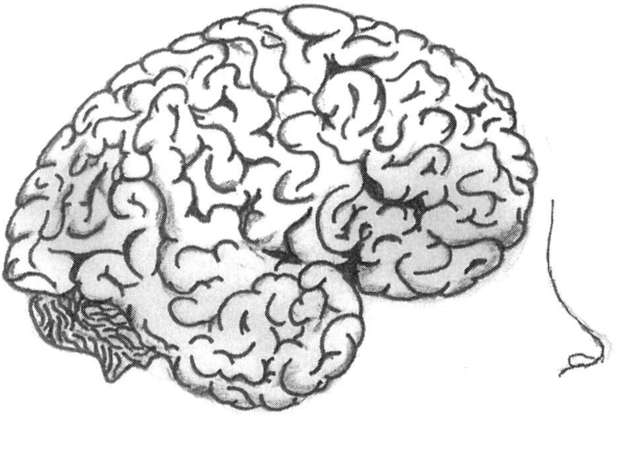

Which parts of the brain can be distinguished?

Broadly speaking, the brain is made up of three parts:

1. central nuclei in the middle (these are also called basal nuclei);
2. the limbic system, which is located between the nuclei and the cortex;
3. the cerebral cortex.

Animals have somewhat similar nuclei in the center, and more advanced animals also have a similar limbic system. The cerebral cortex, on the other hand, is by far the most developed in humans.

What is gray matter?

Gray matter are nerve cells. They are located in the cortex of the brain and in some areas in the middle of the brain. They look gray, both in real life and on a photo taken with an MRI scanner.

What is white matter?

White matter are the long offshoots of nerve cells that connect to cells in other areas of the brain. They are surrounded by a "tube" of myelin. Myelin protects the nerve fibers and accelerates the transport of information. The latter is done via electrical currents. Myelin is a type of insulation that ensures that the current does not leak. Myelin has a white color. Therefore, the nerve fibers look white. These white nerve fibers bundle together and form the "pathways" between the nerve cells that lie in the gray matter regions.

Figure 18.2 Nerve cell

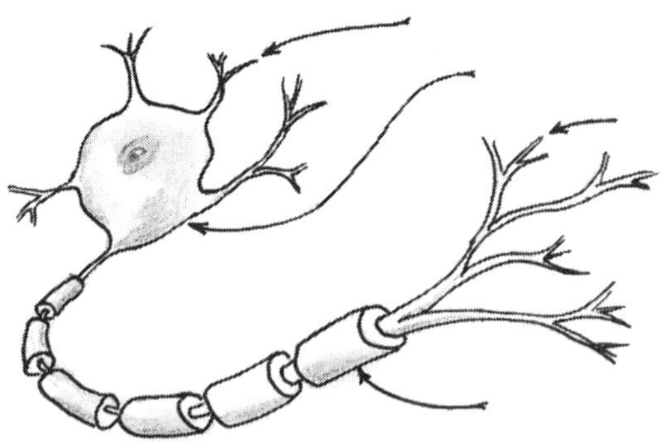

First arrow: receiving nerve fiber; Second arrow: Nerve cell; Third arrow: Outgoing nerve fiber; Fourth arrow: Myelin

What functions do the different brain areas have?

You could compare the nuclei in the middle to a starter motor. Here it is detected whether action is required. If so, things are set in motion. In addition, there is a lot of contact back and forth between nerve cells in the rest of your body and the basal nuclei. How it fares in the rest of your body affects the basal nuclei and vice versa. The action selection that takes place in the basal nuclei is very important: ofcourse you should not react to everything. It would turn you out of control and exhausted. But worse, you would no longer adapt your behavior enough to the people around you. For that reason, there is a strong regulation of the basal nuclei by the cortex and the limbic system. Regulation, in this particular case, means that the cortex and limbic system generally slow down the basal nuclei.

The limbic system processes the information that is important to you emotionally. In parts of the limbic system, important things are stored in your memory (especially in the hippocampus). Moreover, response patterns for social situations are prepared from here. This also concerns many reaction patterns that you have learned in your life.

Specific processing of external stimuli (such as sound, image and feeling) takes place in the cortex. Moreover, motor and social responses are coordinated here. The front part of the gray matter (also called the frontal cortex) is almost continuously busy with guiding your behavior in the right direction. For this reason, an enormous amount of work is put into abating the central nuclei by the cortex.

How can you measure brain volume in someone who is alive?

With MRI (Magnetic Resonance Imaging) you can make an image of the brain. The beauty of a MRI is that no harmful radiation is involved. MRI uses sound waves in a magnetic field to create an image of the body. Due to differences in the water content of different tissue, the shape of those tissues can be depicted. There are no harmful effects of MRI. With a MRI you can distinguish between white matter, gray matter, liquid and bone. By taking several photos, each time from a slightly different level, you can, as it were, make different cross-sections of the brain. This allows you to estimate the volume of the gray matter, white matter and fluid in and around the brain.

Figure 18.3 Different MRI-slices

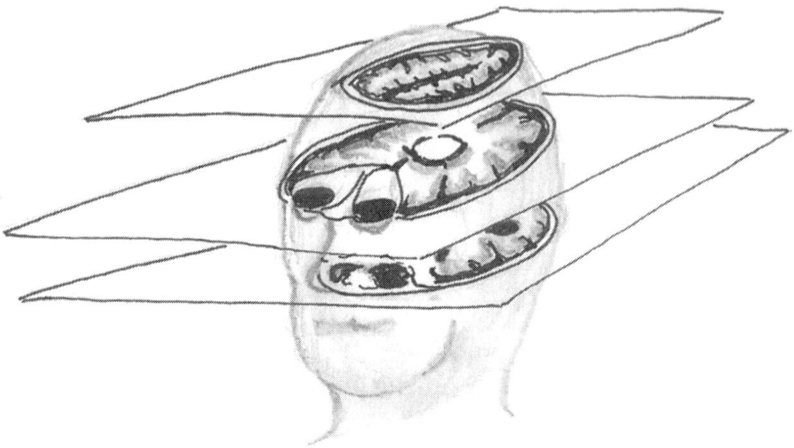

How do brains develop?

The brain's development begins in the womb, but its evolution is also breathtaking in the years that follow. Brains develop on the basis of the challenges that people encounter. That already starts in infancy. There you already learn an incredible amount about your fellow man and about yourself. You learn to look, grasp, listen and laugh. You get to know the effect of your behavior on others. You learn that crying sometimes helps. You learn to understand and speak language. But specific motor systems also develop later in childhood, for example if you play football. In addition, the relationship between what you see and hear and how you respond to it is strongly developed. If you play the piano a lot, you develop the operating system of your fine motor skills, your sense of rhythm and the connection between what you hear and how your fingers move. When you read a lot, you develop the parts of your brain that deal with sense of language, memory and reasoning. Your brain is pre-eminently an organ that can be completely tailored for your life. The fact that the change in the brain is especially impressive during childhood and youth does not mean that nothing happens later in life. The opportunity for change remains, even if it diminishes somewhat in the course of life. But even at the age of 70 you can still learn to paint or tap dance. Maybe not as smooth as when you were eight years old, but you can. Everything you learn is accompanied by changes in your brain. Connections between areas and cells that you use a lot become faster and more efficient, and more connections can also develop. Conversely, if you don't use some of your brain's capabilities, connections become less efficient, weaker and thinner. You can also see this dynamic development in the volume of the brain. An increase in early childhood, then a slight decrease around puberty and up to the age of 45 there is a fairly stable volume.

Between the ages of 12 and 17, the changes in your brain are completely spectacular. This is a phase where there are also significant hormonal changes and puberty manifests in most. You are also vulnerable in that phase. Development can therefore go in an unfavorable direction. We think this is one reason why psychiatric problems usually start in puberty or early adolescence.

What happens with the brain in old age?

Over the years, starting from about the age of 45, brain volume steadily decreases a bit. This is also noticeable in the deterioration of certain brain functions. Older people can compensate for this through their life experience. Some people lose volume faster than others. Smoking is known to cause faster loss of brain tissue. Mental or physical inactivity is also associated with a faster loss of volume. When people stay active in old age, their brains stay in shape longer.

What factors affect brain volume?

The volume of the brain can decrease because unused connections and areas become slimming. You could think of the development of the brain in childhood as sculpting a shape out of a stone. A more lean organization is created that is adapted to the life of that person. This is accompanied by a natural (and healthy) decrease in volume. However, loss of volume can also be caused by inactivity, smoking or excessive or prolonged stress. Physical and sexual abuse and childhood neglect can affect brain development. In later life, the processes that provide nutrition and recovery decrease, so that the volume of brain tissue also decreases.

Are there any indications that, on average, there is more brain volume loss in people with schizophrenia?

There are indications that, on average, there is more brain volume loss in people with schizophrenia. Especially people who meet the classification criteria for schizophrenia at an early age, about thirteen years old, have clearly less brain volume. This trend continues in the first years in which they have the condition. It should be borne in mind that getting schizophrenia at such a young age is very rare and that those children are usually seriously ill. Volume loss has also been shown in people who later develop psychosis for the first time, as well as in people who suffer from a chronic psychosis.

How large is the average loss of volume?

Only recently have studies been published in which patients have been followed for some time. These studies allow us to say something about the course of the loss of brain volume in people with schizophrenia. On average, patients with schizophrenia have 2 percent less gray matter and 1 percent less white matter. The brain volume is on average 1150 milliliters, but in people with schizophrenia the average is 1116 milliliters. It is important to remember that this is an average. Some people with schizophrenia have as much brain tissue as people without schizophrenia. The tissue loss is not due to the loss of cells, but due to a decrease in connections between nerve cells and loss of supporting cells. It is also important to realize that this is a subtle loss of volume and that something can also be done: being active, exercising, eating healthy and not smoking can help! After the first 20 years of the condition, people with schizophrenia do not lose more brain tissue than people without schizophrenia (Van Erp et al. 2015)

Does volume loss also occur in people with other schizophrenia spectrum disorders?

Much less research has been done into volume loss in people with other schizophrenia spectrum disorders. All we know is that even less tissue loss occurs in people with other psychotic conditions than in schizophrenia. In other words, the deviations are even more subtle.

When does that volume loss occur in patients with schizophrenia?

Most studies currently available show that gray matter loss is greatest in the first year of the disease. After that, the gray matter decreases a little faster than in people without schizophrenia, but after the 45th year the volume loss is in line with that of people without schizophrenia. The white matter appears to increase slightly in people with schizophrenia in the period up to the 32nd year of life, and then begin a subtle decline just as in people without schizophrenia.

Is there more volume loss in everyone with schizophrenia than in people without schizophrenia?

As mentioned, everyone loses brain volume from about the age of 45. The increase in loss of brain tissue found was found on average in large groups. However, not everyone with schizophrenia has more volume loss than normal.

Which problems are associated with brain volume loss in people with schizophrenia?

An association has been found between the loss of brain volume and the course of the disease of schizophrenia: if people with schizophrenia recover less well, function less well and have more negative symptoms, there is more loss of brain tissue.

Much research has been done into the influence of antipsychotics on brain volume, but the only study that could provide a definitive answer is ethically irresponsible: randomize people with psychosis to placebo or antipsychotics and then measure brain volume before and after treatment.

We know from animal studies that high doses of antipsychotics lead to brain volume loss. This may be partly due to the inactivity of laboratory animals when they are given a lot of antipsychotics. Research in which the volume of the brain was measured at two times in a large group of patients, shows that the volume decrease is greater in the group taking the highest dose of antipsychotics. Of course, this could be because the people who receive the highest dose also suffer the most from the condition and that the latter factor explains the greater loss of volume. Nevertheless, this finding supports the use of the lowest possible dose of an antipsychotic. On the other hand, it is also important to know that going through another psychosis is associated with about four times the loss of volume as taking antipsychotics for one year.

Cannabis use is associated with increased brain volume loss. It turned out that people who continued to smoke cannabis lost more brain tissue than patients who stopped smoking or had never smoked. The influence of smoking cigarettes is also very clear. The more someone smokes, the greater the decrease in brain volume (Haren et al., 2010).

How does the brain function?

Different parts of the brain work together. The connections that enable this cooperation between brain areas are called the brain network.

What does a brain network have to do with schizophrenia?

Disruptions in the brain network could make it difficult to process information. Disruption of the brain network could also be related to the development of psychotic symptoms.

What does the brain network look like?

On a microscopic level, you can see that the brain is organized as a network of connections between individual brain cells that are connected by synapses. But you can also see that with the naked eye: large bundles of nerve fibers that connect certain parts of the brain. Those bundles of nerve fibers look white, which is why they are called white matter. As you read this text, information travels through your eye to a specific part of the cerebral cortex that processes perceived images (the visual cortex). Then this information goes to a part of the brain that specializes in language processing and to a part that specializes in understanding and remembering.

Figure 18.4 Brain network

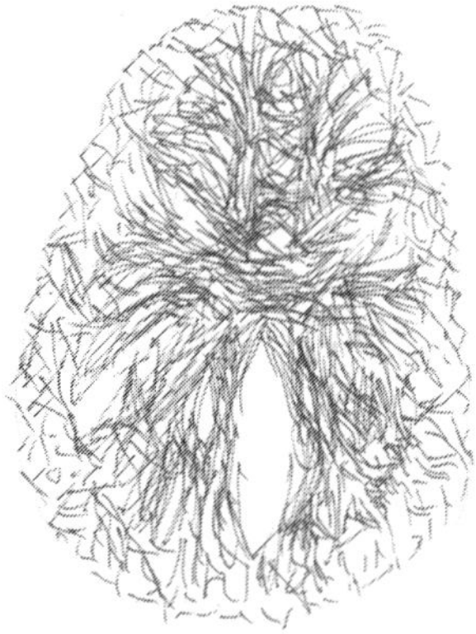

How can you describe the properties of a brain network?

You can describe different characteristics of a network, for example: How many connections go to a certain area; How centrally a certain area is in a network (this is called "centrality"); To what extent certain areas are interconnected (clustering); The length of connections between areas; Whether there are certain groups of areas within networks that are mainly connected to each other (so-called "modules").

What is a functional network?

A functional brain network is a group of areas that are active together during a certain function. For example, when you suddenly perceive sound, areas in which sound stimuli are processed are active along with areas that check whether the perceived sound indicates possible danger. These areas are then active together in a functional network.

Figure 18.5 Central functional organisation

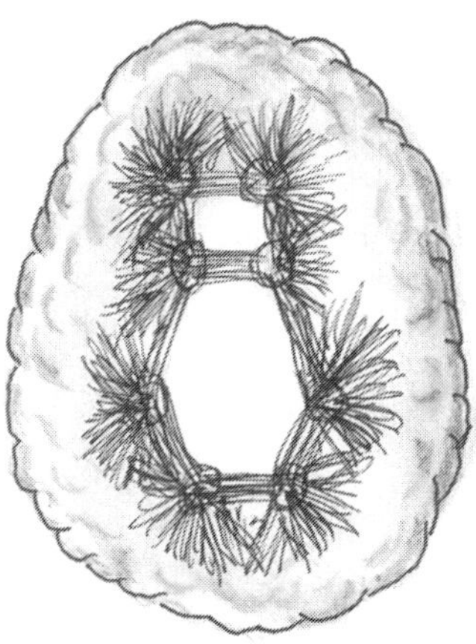

How does a brain network develop?

The main structure of the brain network is already present in newborn babies, but in the first 20 years of life, brain modules continue to develop and the integration of networks increases. Areas that collaborate together are becoming increasingly interconnected, and communication between these areas is progressing faster and faster.

Functional networks in babies are first and foremost concerned with processing images, sound and information about movement and posture. In the course of development, an increasingly large central functional organization is created.

Are there changes in brain networks in people with schizophrenia?

Slightly longer connections are found between areas in people with schizophrenia. That could make information processing a little less efficient. In addition, slightly fewer connections between central areas have been found in people whose problems meet the classification schizophrenia. This could make the central organization of information processing somewhat more difficult. This reduced central network organization is not found in people with bipolar disorder. Functional networks appear to be less clustered in people with schizophrenia. These differences are very subtle (Hulshoff Pol et al. 2004).

Does measuring the brain network tell us something about development or treatment?

There are some studies that indicate that people with schizophrenia in whom antipsychotics do not help have reduced central integration compared to people with schizophrenia in whom the antipsychotics are beneficial. Further research should show whether this finding is useful in practice. Perhaps research on brain networks in the future can contribute to our understanding of the development of vulnerability. Perhaps we will learn how to improve brain networks, although we already know that mental and physical activity helps to keep your brain and brain networks in shape (Peters et al. 2010).

References

Erp, T.G.M. van, Hibar, D.P., Rasmussen, J.M., glahn, D.C., Pearlson, G.D., Andreassen, O.A., e.a. (2015). Subcortical brain volume abnormalities in 2028 individuals with schizophrenia and 2540 healthy controls via the enigma consortium. Molecular Psychiatry, 21(4), 547-553.

Haren, N.E.M. van, Koolschijn, P.C., Cahn, W., Schnack, H.G., Hulshoff Pol, H.E., & Kahn, R.S. (2010). Cigarette smoking and progressive brain volume loss in schizophrenia. European Neuropsychopharmacology, 20(7), 454-458.

Hulshoff Pol, H.E., Schnack, H.G., Mandl, R.C.W., Cahn, W., Collins, D.L.L., Evans, A.C., e.a. (2004). Focal white matter density changes in schizophrenia: reduced inter-hemispheric connectivity. Neuroimag., 21(1), 27-35.

Peters, B.D., Blaas, J., & Haan, L. de (2010). Diffusion tensor imaging in the early phase of schizophrenia: What have we learned? Journal of Psychiatric Research, 44(15), 993-1004.

CHAPTER 19

DOPAMINE AND PSYCHOSIS

Dopamine plays an important role in the theory of the development of psychosis and in the theory of the effect of antipsychotics. Just sit back, because this chapter contains a lot of information.

What is dopamine?

Dopamine is a messenger involved in the transfer of information between nerve cells. Nerve cells form complex networks in the brain with each other. Nerve cells are interconnected by synapses.

Figure 19.1 Synaps

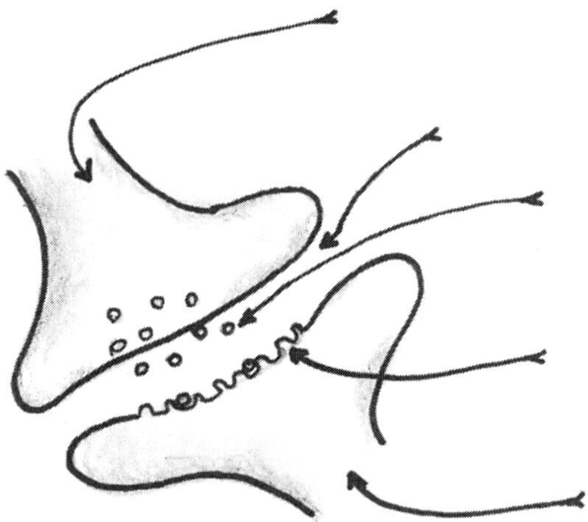

First arrow: incoming nerve fibre; Second arrow: synaps; Third arrow: neurotransmitter, for instance dopamine; Fourth arrow: receptor; Sixth arrow: receiving nerve fibre

Synapses are narrow spaces between nerve cells. When a nerve cell becomes active, messenger substances such as dopamine are released in the synapse. Dopamine travels from the active nerve cell through the synapse to a receiving station of the other nerve cell and attaches to it. This receiving station is called the dopamine receptor. Because dopamine attaches to this receptor, the recipient nerve cell becomes active and can in turn activate other cells. This changes the activity of the network of nerve cells (De Haan, 2018).

What does dopamine do?

Dopamine plays an important role in mental processes such as attention, concentration and learning. In addition, dopamine also plays an important role in movement. Disruption of the functioning of dopamine can therefore cause movement problems. An example of this is Parkinson's disease. In this disease, more than 80 percent of the nerve cells that produce dopamine have been lost. As a result, there is too little dopamine, patients move little and they suffer from stiffness and tremors. This dopamine deficiency can also have psychological consequences: decreased mental flexibility, memory problems and depression.

Figure 19.2

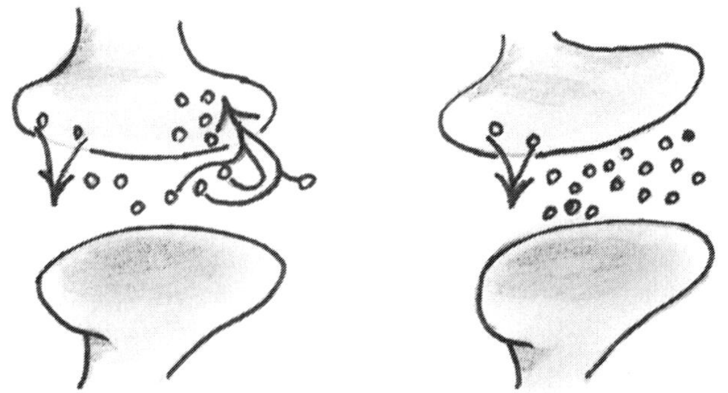

Normally there is reuptake of dopamine | Cocaine prevents reuptake of dopamine

Another example of the influence of dopamine on psychological functioning is the effect of cocaine. Cocaine inhibits dopamine reuptake. Therefore, dopamine stays longer in the synapse and can increasingly occupy and activate the receiving stations of nerve cells, causing more activity in neural networks. This is associated with increased self-confidence, increased alertness and activity, and sometimes with paranoia or other psychotic symptoms (De Haan, 2018).

Is dopamine associated with sex, drugs and rock and roll?

It used to be thought that dopamine only played an important role in pleasurable experiences such as food, music, sex and the use of alcohol and drugs. The idea was: dopamine is increased with sex, drugs and rock and roll. That's right, but it's not the whole story. Dopamine is not only involved in pleasant experiences, but also in unpleasant ones. Moreover, dopamine appears to be released especially when someone expects to have a pleasant experience soon, so before the experience of pleasure. Furthermore, it was found that substances that inhibit the function of dopamine mainly reduce the motivation to make an effort to obtain pleasant experiences, rather than the experience of pleasure itself. That is why it is now believed that dopamine is mainly involved with the importance that a person attaches to experiences or thoughts, both pleasant and unpleasant (Berridge and Robinson, 1998).

What is the relationship between dopamine, importance, motivation and learning?

Attaching importance to something is related to motivation. It can be something you really want or something you are very afraid of. In any case, it is not neutral. Because you attach importance to something, you take action.

For example, if you watch your favorite club play an exciting final on television and a beautiful cross is given, then your dopamine is very active. After all, you expect that very important things are about to happen. You pay very close attention. If someone walks between you and the television, it bothers you and you try to look around him or if you are a little more impulsive, just give him a push.

A very different example: if you walk alone in a dark alley and you know that a few people have been robbed there in recent weeks, then your dopamine is also very active.

In both cases, you pay close attention. You can respond quickly and you remember things well. Dopamine activity increases as soon as something happens that could be important to you. Something you want or something you try to avoid. Or something that is new and unexpected. You could compare dopamine to a highlighter that allows you to make certain passages in a text stand out: this allows events and thoughts to get your full attention. Animals and humans then take purposeful action to obtain or maintain pleasant experiences and to limit or avoid unpleasant experiences. The important new experiences are educational. You can easily remember them because they are important to you (Berridge and Robinson, 1998).

Figure 19.3 Dopamine works like a highlighter

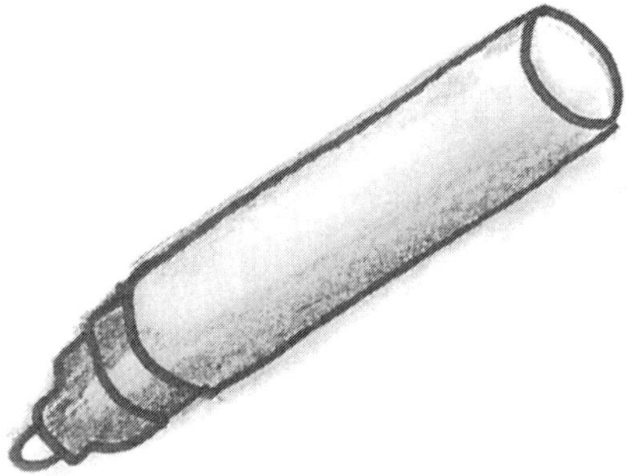

What is the role of dopamine in predicting the future?

Dopamine therefore plays a role in the phase prior to an important event for you. Again, this event can be pleasant or unpleasant and scary. Animals and people try to predict whether they can expect something nice or bad. Because if you can predict what will happen, you can already optimally adjust your behavior. By practicing predicting, you learn how to behave in the best way. Dopamine plays a major role in this prediction. When dopamine is active, the situation you are in is experienced as interesting: you pay more attention, you may be more on your guard and remember better. This ensures that you learn how to experience pleasant things and avoid bad things. In the examples described above, you were already alert and on your guard beforehand. You knew beforehand that something important was about to happen. But dopamine is also released into the synapse if something unexpected happens while you are relaxed. Dopamine release increases when something unpredicted happens. Therefore, the action of dopamine is involved in learning to improve your predictions about the future. Dopamine also rises if your expectation (your prediction) does not come true, if something happens that you had not expected.

Suppose you are on the subway and a young man sits opposite you and smiles at you kindly. His friend sits down next to you. Your expectation is: nice guys, nothing to worry about. You read further in your book. They get off at the next stop and suddenly you notice that your phone is gone. That doesn't match your prediction at all, your dopamine is sky high, you're stressed out. But you also learned something you won't soon forget: not all nice looking guys can be trusted.

The increased dopamine represents the biological side of the signal that something happened that you totally did not expect, and the memories of this event and of your false prediction will remain important to you. In fact, sometimes this event and the memory of it completely change the way you view the world (in other words, your future predictions). For example, you never trust guys who come across as nice again, or you think the subway is always a dangerous place that you should avoid.

A more pleasant example of dopamine's role in false predictions is the following. Suppose you really like someone at a party, but you don't know that person and you are a bit shy. If she comes up to you unexpectedly to have a chat with you, then your dopamine is sky high. You predicted: she doesn't see me at all, but suddenly she turns out to like you too. A prediction error that learned you something: There are people who like me more than I thought.

These properties of dopamine can help us to explain the connection between biological disturbances and symptoms of psychosis. The following paragraphs are about this.

Which theories try to explain the development of the sensitivity to psychosis?

There are two theories that try to explain the development of the sensitivity to psychosis. Those are the dopamine hypothesis and the development hypothesis. Both theories are interrelated.

What is the dopamine hypothesis of psychosis?

The dopamine hypothesis of psychosis was conceived after it was found that antipsychotics work by blocking dopamine receptors (dopamine receiving stations). By blocking dopamine receptors, dopamine cannot activate the recipient nerve cell. In addition, it turned out that substances that stimulate dopamine can actually cause psychotic symptoms. The nature of the dopamine disruption in psychosis was then investigated, as it could be due to various factors. It turned out that most patients who suffer from a psychosis release more dopamine when they experience a stressful situation. It also was found that this increased activity of dopamine persists longer, so that the release of dopamine is increased over a longer period. Later it was also found that dopamine release is higher in patients who are acutely psychotic, and that it decreases again when the severity of the psychosis decreases. No other clear deviations from the "dopamine system" were found. It turned out that there were not more receptors or fewer substances that ensure the removal of dopamine from the synapse (Davis et al. 1991, Howes and Murray 2013, 2017).

Figure 19.4

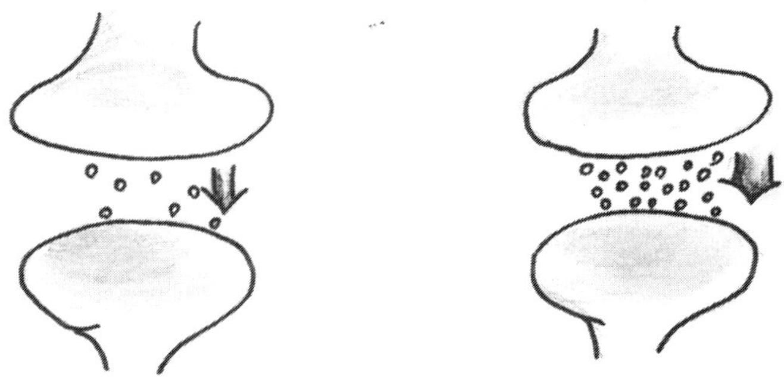

Normal dopamine release

Increased dopamine release during psychosis

What does the developmental hypothesis of schizophrenia spectrum disorders entail?

A developmental hypothesis refers to a theory that explains the emergence of a certain condition from the development in the previous period. The developmental hypothesis of schizophrenia spectrum disorders implies that disturbed development increases the vulnerability to develop psychosis. The developmental hypothesis was conceived because three things stood out in the youth of people who later developed psychosis. In the first place, there appeared to be a connection between certain events before or around childbirth and the risk of developing a schizophrenia spectrum disorder. Second, it was found that in some children who were later diagnosed with schizophrenia in childhood, showed abnormalities in movement, cognitive function or social behavior. Third, there is evidence that subtle changes in the brain are already present during the first phase of schizophrenia spectrum disorder (Davis et al. 1991, Howes and Murray 2013, 2017).

What role does dopamine play in the developmental hypothesis?

Today we think that dopamine also plays an important role in the developmental hypothesis. Animal research has shown that stress during pregnancy or early childhood influence the development of the dopamine system. Inflammation during pregnancy is associated with more dopamine release during stress in adulthood. Oxygen deficiency around birth is also associated with more dopamine release in response to stress during adulthood. But also severe maltreatment (such as sexual abuse) at a young age increase the sensitivity of the dopamine system. Other psychosocial risk factors such as growing up in a large big city or migration also play a role. Moreover, biological risk factors such as cannabis use are also associated with an increased sensitivity and activity of the dopamine system later in life (Howes and Murray 2013, 2017).

How is dopamine related to later development?

In recent years, more evidence has been found for the influence of social risk factors during later development on the risk of developing schizophrenia spectrum disorders. Immigration, growing up in a city, early parental loss and childhood abuse are associated with an approximately doubled chance of developing schizophrenia spectrum disorder (see also Chapter 15 on psychological and social risk factors). From research that repeatedly measures response to daily events, we know that patients with schizophrenia are more sensitive to stress and that even mild stress can cause an increase in psychotic symptoms. Animal studies also show that social isolation during childhood leads to increased dopamine release in response to stress in adulthood. The position in the social hierarchy also appears to have an influence: being the underdog and being at the mercy of major changes in the social environment are associated with increased dopamine release in response to stress.

In humans, the influence of social stressors on the dopamine system has been less researched, because it is not ethical to apply serious social stressors to humans in research. (You may also wonder how ethical it is to do this in laboratory animals.) Research in animals and humans suggests that repeated exposure to stress can cause increased susceptibility to increased dopamine release. You call this sensitization. This can increase your sensitivity to psychosis (Howes and Murray 2013, 2017).

What is the role of dopamine in psychosis?

Briefly, the theory about the relationship between dopamine and psychosis boils down to the following. During a psychosis, dopamine is released to an increased degree. This gives more importance to perceptions, experiences and thoughts. If this condition persists for a long time, people become convinced that something must be wrong, because the perceptions, experiences and thoughts are so impressive. The following example illustrates the psychological consequences of increased dopamine release.

Suppose that you release more dopamine than usual in a somewhat stressful situation and that this increase also persists for a long time. Suppose you have just moved to another city. You walk through the shopping street and everything is still unknown to you. Anyone who experiences this is a little more observant. That is also a great adjustment, because it allows you to learn new things about your new place of residence faster. Dopamine is slightly more active in everyone than in situations with which you are already familiar. But if your dopamine system is extra sensitive, too much dopamine will be released and the increase will persist for a long time. This has consequences for your perceptions, experiences and thoughts. As a result, you can notice while walking that people are all looking at you for a moment. You also see that a few gray cars slow down when they drive next to you. In a "normal" state, these experiences would not impress you, but now it seems very important. The more you notice it, the more you pay attention to how people look at you. Some people don't look at you at all, but you notice that too. Not all gray cars slow down, but the moment you think you might be imagining it, there is another gray car that slows down. It keeps you busy more and more. When you come back to your new home, you still think about it. Could something be wrong? It is so impressive that it is almost impossible that there is nothing behind it? It's so striking. It keeps on going in your head.

If this condition continues for a long time, you can become more and more convinced that something is wrong. At first you doubt whether people in that new city know anything about you or whether the gray cars are slowing down to keep an eye on you. But at some point you know for sure: there is a conspiracy. That idea is of course stressful in itself. But somehow you also feel relieved that you know now, because now you can take precautions. For example, only going out very early, or not going on the streets at all. And no more phone calls, because then they will not be able to hack your cellphone.

How does dopamine relate to what you experience and think?

Because more dopamine is released, it seems that everyday observations or thoughts are very important. It is simply the case that many people in a shopping street take a look at you. But it's not that important, and in a normal situation you don't pay much attention to it or think about it either. The same is true of seeing cars slowing down, as well as the thought that your phone could be hacked. That can indeed happen, but normally you are not so concerned with it. But because dopamine is released at an increased rate, you continue to notice it, you keep paying attention and at a certain point you cannot think about anything else. If dopamine then stays at an elevated level for a long time, these experiences and thoughts seem super important, and at some point you become convinced that you are in danger and that you need to be on your guard.

Later on, people who developed psychosis say about this pre-psychosis phase: "I became more aware of what was going on around me. It was as if my senses became more sensitive. I was fascinated by the trifles in my environment. Or," What I saw and heard had a clarity that I had never experienced before". They get the idea that something has changed in the world around them, making them feel anxious and overwhelmed. During the course of this preliminary phase, which can last from days to years, people have impressions that seem abnormally important and for which they have no explanation at the time (De Haan, 2018).

How do delusions arise?

When there is a significant increase in dopamine, and especially if the increase continues for a long time, people can develop ideas of their own that explain the things they perceive or experience. If those ideas are clearly unrealistic and the patient is the only one who is convinced of the truth and his or her conviction cannot be changed, then these ideas are called delusions. So, delusions are beliefs or thoughts that arise in order to give meaning to the impressive experiences that seem so important. Once someone has found an explanation for those important experiences and thoughts, relief may set in. From that moment on, the delusion acts as a guiding scheme for future thoughts and actions.

How do hallucinations arise?

Hallucinations can also occur with psychosis. Hallucinations are, for example, hearing voices when no one in the outside world is speaking to you. How should you understand the link between hallucinations and dopamine? Due to a high level of dopamine, you attach more importance to memories or internal speech. The memory or internal speech is more noticeable and more impressive. The importance attached to memories or internal speech may also be related to the different manifestations of hallucinations. These can vary from amplified own thoughts and hearing your own voice to hearing the voice of others. An increased dopamine level also appears to influence the detection of the origin of observations. Due to the increased release of dopamine, you are less able to determine whether something you experience comes from within or from outside.

However, the explanation of hallucinations due to increased dopamine release is less convincing than the link between dopamine and delusions. Another mechanism is likely to be involved in hallucinations. Normally, when you think or speak, the sensitivity of the center in your brain that processes sound is inhibited. In people who have acoustic hallucinations, this inhibition is not optimal. This allows you to experience that you hear something while you think. Under the influence of an increased dopamine release you will attach more importance to these special observations (De Haan, 2018).

What happens when the increased dopamine release decreases?

If the level of dopamine decreases, then the severity of psychosis decreases. It is often striking that it is not so much the content of people's beliefs that changes, as the importance they attach to them. A similar process occurs in reducing hallucinations. The volume of the hallucinations and the frequency with which they occur decrease during recovery. It is not so much the message of the voices that changes. Even the belief that voices come from outside often persists. However, the impact of the voices gradually diminishes: they make less impression and disappear from the center of attention (De Haan, 2018).

What is a Fundamental Property of Antipsychotics?

Substances that inhibit the action of dopamine reduce the importance attached to an experience and the impact of an experience on behavior. So, animals and people become more indifferent to experiences. It hurts them less. This is the fundamental property that all antipsychotics share. When patients who suffer from delusions take antipsychotics, the effect of dopamine decreases, reducing the importance they attach to these experiences and ideas. Likewise, antipsychotics reduce the importance attached to hallucinations.

The importance of ideas and perceptions diminishes, making people feel calmer (Kapur, 2003).

Figure 19.5

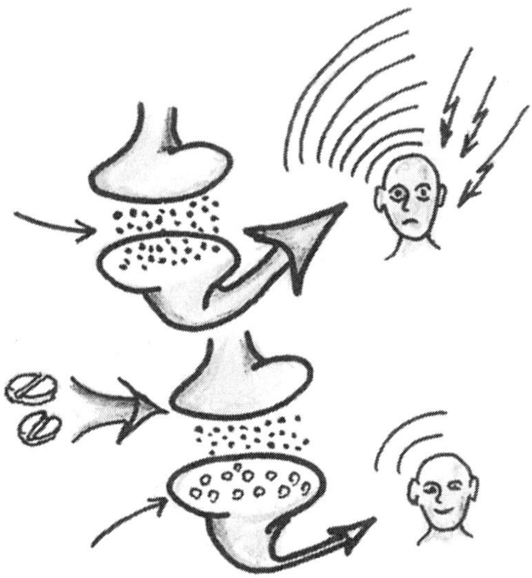

First arrow: Increased release of dopamine activates dopamine receptors; Second arrow: Antipsychotic drugs occupy the dopamine receptor and therefore dopamine can not activate these receptors

How Do Antipsychotics Work?

One theory of the mechanism of action of antipsychotics explains the effects of antipsychotic treatment. Antipsychotics block the dopamine receptor. They sit on that receptor, which prevents dopamine from transmitting its message. Dopamine blockade develops very quickly after the first administration of antipsychotics, and consequently the severity of psychotic symptoms decreases rapidly. Especially the importance attached to delusions diminishes.

Often it turns out that people continue to believe in the ideas they had, but these thoughts are no longer so important to them because of the antipsychotics. You may wonder why people continue to believe their delusions. This probably has to do with people not changing their minds quickly. Certainly, if you have had a thought that is important to you for a long time and with conviction, there is a tendency to stick to it. That's not to say the antipsychotics aren't doing their job. What matters in the treatment with antipsychotics is that people no longer suffer from a certain belief, that the delusion is no longer in the foreground and that there develops room to pay attention to other matters.

As mentioned, antipsychotics block the dopamine receptor, but do not inhibit dopamine production. The amount of dopamine produced may even increase at the beginning of the treatment. However, because the dopamine receptors are blocked, the released dopamine no longer has any effect. Dopamine released in the space between nerve cells is reabsorbed into the producing cell and reused.

The dampening effect of antipsychotics does not only affect experiences and thoughts that are given too much importance. Especially when the dosage of an antipsychotic is too high, all thoughts and experiences become less important. Then patients complain of flattening or an unpleasant feeling: the effect of dopamine is then too much inhibited. The sense of flattening is the flipside of the fundamental mechanism of antipsychotics: dampening the degree of importance attached to the experience. It helps to diminish heightened meaning making and overly impressive experiences, but attaching importance to perceptions and ideas is also the driving force behind human activities and interactions.

If experiences become too flat, it is wise to consult your psychiatrist to seek a lower dose or an antipsychotic that has less adhesion to the dopamine receptor. The sensitivity to antipsychotics can vary from person to person and is related to the individual characteristics of the dopamine system. That is why tailor-made work is necessary and the lowest possible effective dosage must always be sought in the treatment of psychosis: sufficient to reduce delusions, hallucinations or confusion, but at the same time so little that normal motivation hardly suffers (De Haan, 2018).

Figure 19.6

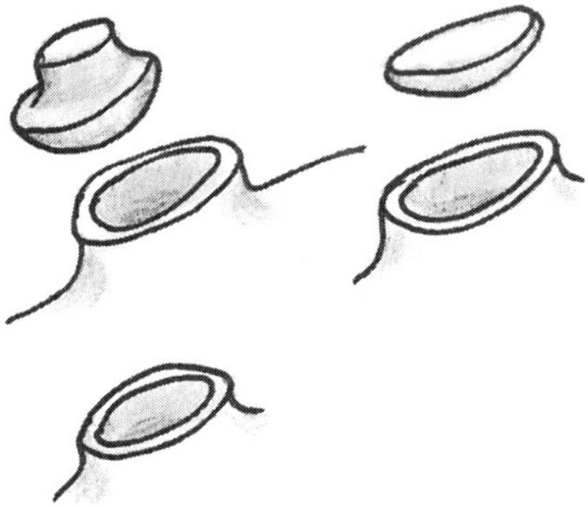

Antipsychotic medication and dopamine both are able to occupy the dopamine receptor. When antipsychotic medication occupies the dopamine receptor, then this receptor can not be activated by dopamine (Kapur, 2003).

Why should treatment with antipsychotics be tailor-made?

There are indications that there is an optimal dopamine level: excessive release of dopamine causes anxiety and can be very unpleasant, but too little dopamine production causes flattening. People with psychosis also differ greatly in their dopamine system. As a result, the effects of antipsychotics also differ between people. What is too high a dose for one person is insufficient for another. It is necessary to look for an individual dose offering an optimal level of dopamine action. That is often quite a task. We cannot predict for whom which antipsychotic in which dosage is optimal. Often psychotic experiences still remain. It is always needed to try to find the right balance between effect and side effects (De Haan et al. 2000, 2003).

Do antipsychotics that inhibit dopamine always have a beneficial effect?

Antipsychotics that inhibit dopamine do not always work. In about 25 to 30 percent of patients with a first psychosis, the usual antipsychotics have little or no effect on the psychotic symptoms. It is not exactly clear how this comes about. However, there are research findings that point to the following. People whose psychosis does not improve during antipsychotic treatment have not been found to have a markedly increased release of dopamine. This could explain the lack of effect of antipsychotics. After all, if the dopamine is not increased, inhibiting it does not help.

So, 25 to 30 % of the patients suffer from psychosis without a clear dopamine increase. Apparently, dysregulation other neurotransmitter systems than increased dopamine release can also be associated with psychosis. Maybe dopamine is dysregulated, maybe other neurotransmitters are abnormal. Clozapine does have a good effect on psychosis in about 50 percent of patients in whom regular antipsychotics do not help. Clozapine blocks the dopamine receptor in a much less robust way and acts on other neurotransmitters as well. It may therefore be more effective in people with psychosis without a clear increase in dopamine.

What good is the dopamine theory in psychotherapy?

Antipsychotics do not make psychotic symptoms disappear. They reduce the importance attached to delusions and hallucinations, making patients better able to focus on other issues. This creates space to develop other thoughts and views. This process is very similar to the way people gradually distance themselves from long-held beliefs or fears. People generally have a lot of trouble adjusting beliefs, let alone putting them behind them completely.

The increased release of dopamine acts as a driving force, but memories, personal history and social and cultural context determine the content of the psychosis. It follows that specific psychotherapy for psychosis could complement the effect of antipsychotics. The usual treatment for psychosis usually consists of antipsychotics that affect biological processes. Often less attention is paid to specific psychotherapeutic interventions to influence psychotic thoughts and to arrive at new and more appropriate explanations or beliefs. This may help some patients to find more balance. On the other hand, it is also increasingly recognized that it is helpful to pay attention to the things you value in life. When you focus on your friends, loved-ones, work and all the things you feel commitment for, then it helps to decrease the importance of delusions.

The dopamine theory thus provides an explanation for the connection between biological phenomena in the brain and the personal experience of psychosis. It can thus help patients to better understand the overwhelming experience of psychosis. Knowing that may reinforce the sense of self-control. The theory emphasizes that patients do not have to be a plaything of the condition. Instead, it is emphasized that reducing stress and regaining control and self-confidence can break the vicious circle caused by increased dopamine levels (Kapur, 2003).

What are limitations of the dopamine theory of psychosis?

The dopamine theory does not provide a conclusive explanation for the development of schizophrenia spectrum disorders. The theory mainly describes how psychotic symptoms are associated with increased dopamine activity. The theory also applies to other conditions involving psychotic symptoms.

In this chapter, the relationship between the effect of dopamine and other symptoms that occur in schizophrenia spectrum disorders has not been elaborated. It is quite conceivable that disruption of the functioning of dopamine can give rise to experiences that are too important (psychotic symptoms or positive symptoms). The relationship between dopamine and cognitive or motivational problems has not been discussed in this chapter. Animal research has shown that an increase in dopamine can hinder learning through rewarding stimuli. On the other hand, it is also the case that excessive inhibition of dopamine action by antipsychotics can actually amplify negative symptoms and reduce the motivation to take action.

A major limitation of the dopamine theory of psychosis is that elevated levels of dopamine have not been found in all patients who suffer from psychosis. More dopamine release is likely to explain the psychotic symptoms for the majority of patients, but not for all patients.

Dopamine, in short?

In this chapter a theory of psychosis is discussed in which biological, causal, pharmacological and psychotherapeutic aspects are integrated. Dopamine plays a central role in the extent to which importance is attached to experiences, perceptions and thoughts. When dopamine is released at an increased rate, more importance is attached to experiences and thoughts. Delusions are attempts to give meaning to experiences and thoughts that have acquired increased importance. Hallucinations are partly the result of an increase in the importance placed on memories and internal speech. Antipsychotics dampen the importance attached to symptoms, making psychotic symptoms less meaningful.

The dopamine development hypothesis boils down to the following. Genetic variation in interaction with environmental influences in early childhood allows a more sensitive dopamine system to develop. Under the influence of unfavorable or stressful environmental factors during later development, an excessive and longer lasting dopamine release occurs in response to stress. This ensures that extra importance is assigned to neutral experiences or thoughts. This can lead to false beliefs and/or a disturbed perception. This can subsequently cause more stress and lead to less contact with others, causing psychotic beliefs to further increase (Kapur, 2003).

References

Berridge, K.C., & Robinson, T.E. (1998). What is the role of da in reward: Hedonic impact, reward learning, or incentive salience? Brain Res Brain Res Rev, 28(3), 309-369.

Davis, K.L., Kahn, R.S., Ko, G., & Davidson, M. (1991). da in schizophrenia: A review and reconceptualization. Am J Psychiatry, 148(11), 1474-1486.

De Haan Lieuwe. 2018. "Dopamine en Importantie" In Handboek schizofreniespectrumstoornissen, edited by Wiepke Cahn, Inez Myin-Germeys, Richard Bruggeman, Lieuwe de Haan. Amsterdam: De Tijdstroom.

Haan, L. de, Bruggen, M. van, Lavalaye, J., Booij, J., Dingemans, P., & Linszen, D. (2003). Subjective experience and D2 receptor occupancy in patients with schizophrenia, treated with low dose olanzapine or haloperidol: A randomized double-blind study Am J Psychiatry, 160,303-309.

Haan, L. de, Lavalaye, J., Linszen, D.H., Dingemans, P.M.A.J., & Booij, J. (2000). Subjective experience and striatal da D2 receptor occupancy in patients with schizophrenia stabilized on olanzapine or risperidone. Am J Psychiatry, 157, 1019-1020.

Howes, O.D., & Murray, R.M. (2014). Schizophrenia: an integrated sociodevelopmental-cognitive model. Lancet, 383(9929), 1677-1687.

Howes, O.D., McCutcheon, R., Owen, M.J., & Murray, R.M. (2017). The role of genes, stress, and dopamine in the development of schizophrenia. Biol Psychiatry, 81(1), 9-20.

Kapur, S. (2003). Psychosis as a state of aberrant salience: A framework linking biology, phenomenology and pharmacology in schizophrenia. Am J Psychiatry, 160(1), 13-23.

Mizrahi, R., Rusjan, P., Agid, O., Graff, A., Mamo, D.C., Zipursky, RB., e.a. (2007). Adverse subjective experience with antipsychotics and its relationship to striatal and extrastriatal D-2 receptors: A pet study in schizophrenia. Am J Psychiatry, 164, 630-637.

CHAPTER 20

GLUTAMATE

What is glutamate and what does it do?

Glutamate is an amino acid, a building block for proteins. Glutamate is found in all cells of the body. It is also the main activating messenger in the central nervous system. A messenger is a substance involved in transferring information from one nerve cell to another. Glutamate can be expelled from an active nerve cell into the synapse, after which it can be taken up by the next nerve cell or supporting glial cell. There are several glutamate receptors that, when occupied by glutamate, can pass ions, causing electrical changes in the nerve cell. This makes the nerve cell active.

Glutamate abnormalities are thought to contribute to brain tissue loss. This is explained below (Marsman and Hulshoff Pol, 2018).

What does the NMDA receptor have to do with schizophrenia?

A certain type of glutamate receptor, called the NMDA receptor, is involved in the brain's ability to adapt (also known as plasticity). There are indications that the NMDA receptors work slightly less well in people with schizophrenia. This is thought because substances that reduce the function of the NMDA receptor (for example ketamine) cause negative symptoms and psychotic symptoms. Reduced action of the NMDA receptors inhibits the action of GABA, another messenger. GABA is involved in reducing activity. Less effect of GABA causes increased stimulation. The body tries to compensate for the less well-functioning of the NMDA receptor by producing higher levels of glutamate. This is an attempt to improve the functioning of the NMDA receptor. But a high concentration of glutamate can cause nerve cell damage or even loss of nerve cells. This is the mechanism by which too much glutamate may contribute to brain tissue loss. In schizophrenia, an increased concentration of glutamate has been found in the nuclei in the center of the brain. In other areas of the brain, a decrease in glutamate has been discovered.

Many studies of brain tissue and cerebrospinal fluid, as well as large-scale genetic research, indicate that glutamate and reduced NMDA receptor function play a role in the development of vulnerability to schizophrenia. But it is complicated stuff, there are many more types of glutamate receptors. Research into this is underway (Marsman and Hulshoff Pol, 2018).

Can we treat glutamate abnormalities?

Much research has been done into substances that can influence the effect of glutamate. Studies show mixed results: some symptoms improved and some did not. Nevertheless, a meta-analysis (combining 26 studies) found that substances that affect the glutamate system (such as at least four weeks of treatment with the following four different substances: D-serine, glycine, D-cycloserine or D-alanine) cause limited improvement in positive, negative, and cognitive symptoms. Further research is underway (Marsman and Hulshoff Pol, 2018).

References

Marsman Anouk, Hulshoff Pol Hilleke. 2018. "Glutamaterge neurotransmissie" In Handboek schizofreniespectrumstoornissen, edited by Wiepke Cahn, Inez Myin-Germeys, Richard Bruggeman, Lieuwe de Haan. Amsterdam: De Tijdstroom.

CHAPTER 21

STRESS

What is Stress?

Studying for an exam, worrying about the size of your ears, being in love, cutting your fingers, being chased by a criminal, choosing your wedding dress, organizing a party, arguing at school ... Stress comes in many guises.

With stress there is always a stressor that puts you out of balance. This imbalance automatically triggers a response aimed at restoring balance: the stress response. This stress response is very important to your survival. Because of the stress response (and the stress hormones) you pay more attention, you can run faster and react faster, and you feel less pain. It is a response to threatening situations that allows people to react immediately to prevent further damage.

What can be the consequences of chronic stress?

If the stress persists for a long time or comes back again and again, the persistent stress response is harmful to your body and your psychological functioning. Possible consequences are damage to the heart and blood vessels, unfavorable changes in your metabolism and immune system, and an increased inflammatory tendency. Your confidence in a positive outcome or even in yourself or in your fellow human beings can also decrease due to chronic stress. Virtually all psychiatric conditions, including psychosis, are associated with stress.

What is the biology of the stress response like?

Humans and animals have two biological stress systems. First, the sympathetic adrenal medulla system. In the blink of an eye, the adrenal medulla in response to the stressor injects hormones into your blood that activate your sympathetic nervous system. The sympathetic nervous system prepares you for action: your heart beats faster, you breathe faster, and less blood goes to your stomach and more to your muscles and brain.

You can notice this when you suddenly have to do something exciting. Suddenly, you bump into the girl you've been secretly in love with for ages. Your heart is pounding in your throat. You feel a knot in your stomach [or butterflys…].

Second, there is a slower system involving the hypothalamus, pituitary and adrenal cortex. Cortisol is released from the adrenal cortex. This slower system is mainly aimed at adapting the body to the stress and recovery.

Figure 21.1 Stress system

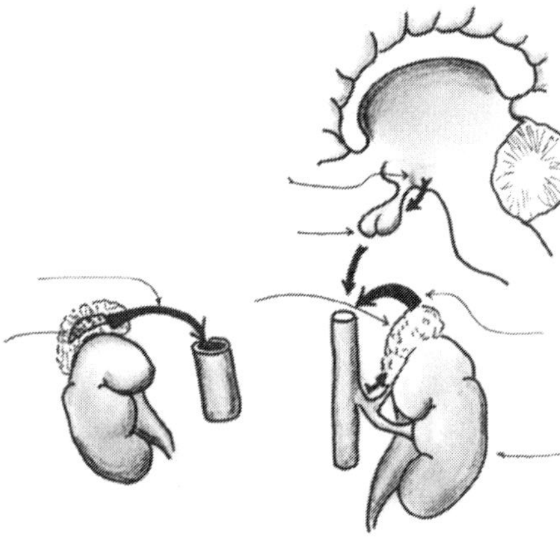

First arrow left: adrenaline; Second arrow left: adrenal medulla; First arrow middle: hypothalamus; Second arrow middle: hypofyse; Third arrow middle: adrenal cortex; First arrow right: cortisol; Second arrow right: kidney

Is stress a risk factor for psychosis?

Some people are more sensitive to stress and stress may induce more and more persistent dopamine release in these individuals. Also, an increasing sensitivity to repetitive stressful situations could play a role. From that perspective, it is not inconceivable that minor, everyday stressors are involved in the development or persistence of psychosis. The latter mechanism is called sensitization. Sensitization means that people continue to respond equally strongly to a milder stressor or that they respond more and more strongly to the same stressor.

For example, you got up too late. Because of this you have to hurry. During breakfast you knock over the milk. That too. You quickly clean up the mess and leave for work, full of stress. Then there is also a subway out. Normally this is already annoying, but now you cannot cope with it. You are very nervous and cranky.

If you come to work in this state and a co-worker criticizes you, you get angry. All of the previous minor irritations have diminished your ability to respond in a balanced way. You are more sensitive to stress now.

What biological mechanisms of stress sensitivity are there in people with psychosis?

Cortisol rises when people experience chronic stress. If cortisol rises, for example because it is given as a medicine or because it is increased in certain diseases, psychotic symptoms can develop. In people with a first psychosis, we find less cortisol emissions in response to stress. Perhaps this is a compensation mechanism for previous hyperactivity. But dopamine also plays a role. A markedly increased level of dopamine breakdown products after stress has been found in psychotic patients, as in people at an increased risk of psychosis and to a lesser extent also in relatives of patients with schizophrenia. This response was also found in response to relatively small daily stressors. If more dopamine breakdown products are found, this means that more dopamine has been released in the preceding period (Vaessen and Myin-Germeys, 2018).

Are there changes in the brain due to stress in people with psychosis?

An enlargement of the pituitary gland has been found in people with a high risk of developing a psychosis and in people who are at the beginning of a first psychosis. This may indicate a chronic stress response and sensitization. In people with psychosis, a correlation was also found between the size of the pituitary gland and the strength of the stress response. Children with an increased risk of psychosis do not yet have an enlarged pituitary gland. Perhaps sensitization has not yet begun.

Long-term elevated cortisol levels can decrease the volume of a particular brain area, the hippocampus. The hippocampus is involved in memory and learning, as well as in the stress response. Childhood trauma and recent stress can also decrease the volume of the hippocampus. Damage to the hippocampus can occur when someone is exposed to excessive stress for a long time. It has been found that during treatment with antipsychotics, the volume of the hippocampus increases again (Vaessen and Myin-Germeys, 2018).

Have other changes in the stress response been found?

In a single study, it was found that parasympathetic nervous system activity is decreased in patients with schizophrenia and, to a lesser extent, in their first-degree relatives. The parasympathetic nervous system is about rest and restoring. If the parasympathetic nervous system is less active, recovery from a stress response may be slower (Vaessen and Myin-Germeys, 2018).

Are there forms of psychotherapy to reduce stress?

Dealing with stressors is central to new forms of behavioral therapy. It is precisely trying to avoid negative experiences that is associated with high stress levels. Fighting thoughts or fears doesn't help: it actually makes thoughts and fears bigger because you pay so much attention to them. It is precisely when you can accept difficulties that your focus on those difficulties diminishes, so that they start to bother you less. That's why it's important to practice accepting things you are concerned about. Therapies such as Acceptance and Commitment Therapy may have a beneficial effect on this (see also Chapter 42 on psychotherapy).

For example, you are afraid of making a mistake when you have to give a presentation in your school. Because you want to prevent that at all costs, you prepare very well. That in itself is fine, but you go further. You are so afraid that you will say something wrong or that you will not be able to get your words out that you memorize the presentation completely. As a result, you have lost your spontaneity. You rattle your story and what you were already afraid of happens: your classmates don't think your story is that good and a bit boring. You notice that, and because of that you actually become even more tense and you become even less spontaneous.

A start to a solution to this problem is to accept that you can make a fool of yourself, or that you may not be able to get out of your words or start to stutter. All of that can happen, but so what? How bad is it when people laugh at you? If you can accept that you are making mistakes and realize that it isn't the end of the world then you can relax more, telling your story more spontaneously and more vividly.

References

Vaessen Thomas, Myin-Germeys Inez. 2018. "Stress" In Handboek schizofreniespectrumstoornissen, edited by Wiepke Cahn, Inez Myin-Germeys, Richard Bruggeman, Lieuwe de Haan. Amsterdam: De Tijdstroom.

CHAPTER 22

NEUROPHYSIOLOGY

What problems can patients with schizophrenia spectrum disorder have with processing information?

Patients with a schizophrenia spectrum disorder can be more sensitive to environmental stimuli. People with schizophrenia can experience too many stimuli at a party or on a busy street. Furthermore, it may be more difficult for them to concentrate or to remember something. Also, sometimes patients cannot distance themselves from certain beliefs. The biological side of information processing is investigated with neurophysiological research. We know that sensitivity to stimuli plays a role in psychotic disorders.

What has electricity to do with information processing?

Transfer of information in the nervous system occurs through electrical activity of nerve cells. Tiny electrical currents travel along the nerve fibers to other nerve cells. This continuous electrical activity of the brain can be measured by electrodes on the outside of scalp. You call this an electroencephalogram (EEG).

How is the EEG used in research into information processing?

When you give someone a certain stimulus (for example suddenly let her hear a sound), activity arises in the brain. The electrical activity in response to this stimulus can be measured on the skull. You will then see certain wave patterns.

Figure 22.1 EEG

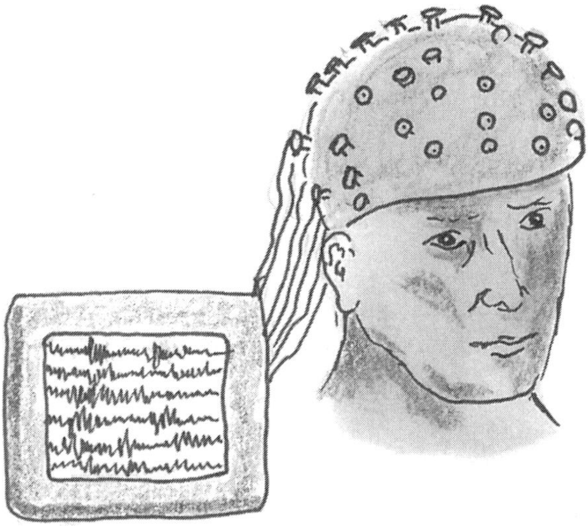

How does the brain prevent overstimulation?

Our brains are constantly bombarded with information. That is why it is necessary to filter out unnecessary stimuli. An example of filtering stimuli is the following. Suppose you hear two loud noises in succession. A lot of activity is generated at the first loud noise. With the second loud noise, that activity is less. You have heard the sound before and are less shocked by it. Information processing is inhibited. That happens unconsciously.

It is also possible that a repeating sound makes you anxious, but that only happens if you think that this sound is related to something dangerous. Then the unconscious filter no longer works. Because you think the sound might be dangerous, you start paying more and more attention (Nieman and Van Tricht Mirjam, 2018).

Are there neurophysiological indications that this filter works less well in people with schizophrenia?

Patients with schizophrenia have a less inhibited response to the second loud sound. So, stimuli continue to have more of an impact. Repetitive stimuli are less well damped or filtered in individuals with schizophrenia.

Are there any indications that a change in stimuli is less easily detected in people with schizophrenia?

If you let people hear a monotonous sound and suddenly something changes in it, then you see that as a reaction in the EEG. This response is less marked in people with schizophrenia. Apparently, the monotonous sound already makes such an impression that the change is less noticeable to them.

Are there any indications that conscious information processing is different in people with schizophrenia?

If you ask people to press a button when they suddenly hear a different tone, you can measure the conscious information processing. Although people with schizophrenia generally do this just as well as people without schizophrenia, EEG research shows that it takes a little longer for patients to process the most important information and that the amount of activity is slightly less. This is also found in relatives of people with schizophrenia.

You can also ask people to look exactly the other way from a moving point of light. That is a difficult task because you have a strong tendency to look at something that moves, so you have to suppress this knee-jerk reaction. This task is difficult for everyone, but people with schizophrenia have a little more difficulty with this task than others.

In addition, some of the patients with schizophrenia are less able to keep following a moving object with their eyes. They sometimes lose the object for a moment and then catch up to get it back into view (Nieman and Van Tricht Mirjam, 2018).

Why is neurophysiological research in people with schizophrenia important?

Patients with schizophrenia spectrum disorders have varying degrees of difficulty processing information. This can affect a person's ability to process stimuli from the environment. The rapid processing of information is of great importance for education, work and social contact. If you process information a little bit more slowly, you may experience new information, as you are still processing previous input. This makes you feel overloaded. However, the variation in the group of people with schizophrenia is very large. Just like the variation among people without schizophrenia, by the way. In the future, neurophysiological studies may be able to help distinguish groups of patients who need additional treatment. It is also being investigated whether neurophysiological characteristics can help predict the risk of developing psychosis (Nieman and Van Tricht Mirjam, 2018).

References

Nieman Dorien, Van Tricht Mirjam. 2018. "Neurofysiologie" In Handboek schizofreniespectrumstoornissen, edited by Wiepke Cahn, Inez Myin-Germeys, Richard Bruggeman, Lieuwe de Haan. Amsterdam: De Tijdstroom.

CHAPTER 23

IMMUNE SYSTEM

What does the immune system do?

The immune system protects the body against infections with parasites, fungi, viruses and bacteria. These organisms are named pathogens. Furthermore, the immune system also protects against disrupted body cells and is involved in recovery after damage has occurred. To do this properly, the immune system must be able to recognize parasites, fungi, viruses, bacteria, disrupted body cells and tissue damage. The big problem with the corona pandemic was that the human body was not yet aware of the virus COVID-19 and that no one's immune system was prepared for it, so the infection could have serious consequences.

The immune system is a defense system. It is important that it is sufficiently active, but also that it responds appropriately. Not too weak, but not too strong either.

Figure 23.1 Defense against virus, bacteria, fungi, deranged cells

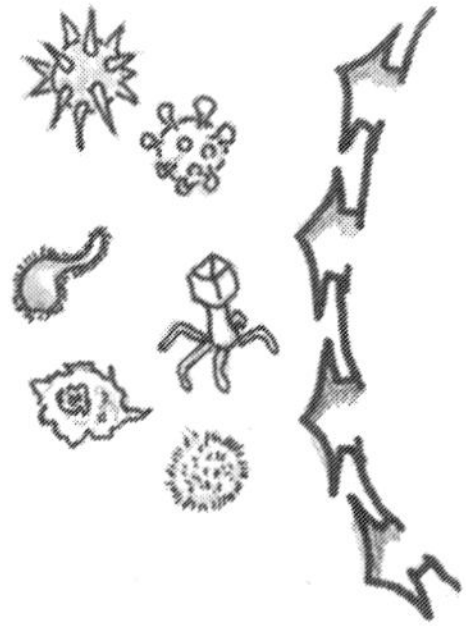

What is the innate immune system and what does it do?

The innate immune system consists of cells (for example granulocytes, monocytes and macrophages) and produces the first acute immune response when a pathogen or harmful stimulus is detected. In addition, it ensures the start of the adaptive immune system.

Figure 23.2

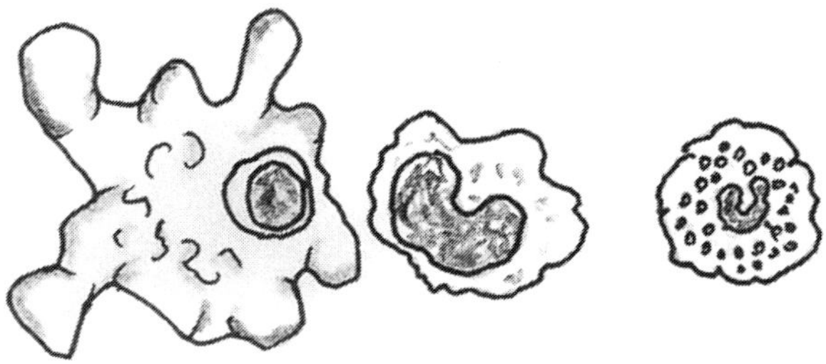

Macrofage Monocyte Granulocyte

What is the adaptive immune system and what does it do?

The adaptive immune system also consists of cells (for example lymphocytes) that produce antibodies that are precisely aimed at a specific pathogen or harmful stimulus. The adaptive system learns from previous contact with pathogens and can respond quickly if a particular pathogen has been identified previously. That way, the body learns to attack pathogens and prevent infections. The coronavirus has caused serious illness in some people because the virus was unknown. We had no antibodies against it yet, because we never encountered that virus before. How the immune system reacts varies from person to person. We also see that with the corona virus: some people become critically ill, others hardly notice the infection.

Figure 23.3 Adaptive immune system

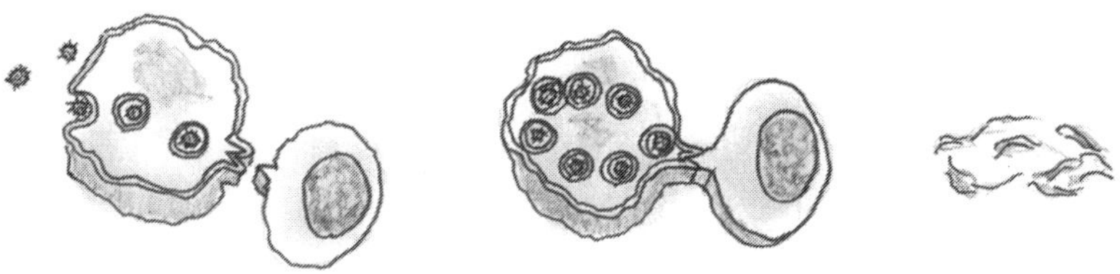

Antigen signals that cell is infected

Adaptive lymphocyte binds to infected cell and develops antibodies

Infected cell and virus destroyed

What is the role of the immune system in the brain?

There are cells in the brain that belong to the innate immune system (for example microglia). Microglia are not only involved in inflammation, but also in the development of synapses and the removal of synapses that are not functioning properly.

Figure 24.4 Microglia attached to nerve cell

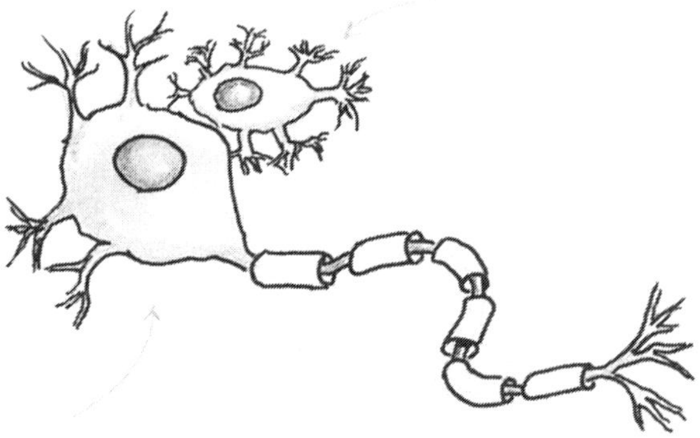

What can go wrong with the immune system?

Sometimes the immune system does not respond or reacts too slowly to pathogens or other harmful stimuli. This is the case, for example, with AIDS, which can cause infections and cancers.

Sometimes the immune system reacts too quickly or too strongly. This is the case, for example, with allergies such as hay fever or a reaction to your own healthy cells (this is called an autoimmune disorder). The inflammation can also last too long, such as with certain intestinal diseases. Excessive immune activity puts stress on the body and can cause damage.

Why do we think the immune system has something to do with schizophrenia?

An important argument is that a link has been found between infections with viruses in the mother or the toxoplasma parasite and the risk of schizophrenia. Other autoimmune conditions such as celiac disease or psoriasis are more common in patients with schizophrenia. On the other hand, rheumatism is less common in them, while it is also an autoimmune disease. Genetic variation associated with the immune system is also found in patients with schizophrenia. Finally, an indirect argument for immune system involvement in schizophrenia is that some antipsychotics have a regulatory influence on the immune system (Van Mierlo and De Witte, 2018).

Which biological findings indicate immune system involvement in schizophrenia?

Large genetic studies have shown that some of the genetic variation associated with schizophrenia is also related to the immune system. More T lymphocytes have also been found in patients with a first psychosis who have never used antipsychotics. More inflammatory factors were found in the blood in patients with current psychosis. This diminished when the psychosis decreased. In addition, a certain protein involved in inflammation (C-reactive protein or CRP) is found to an increased extent in the blood of patients with schizophrenia. A small minority (probably much less than 3 percent) of the patients have antibodies against the NMDA receptor. Finally, increased microglial cell activation was seen in patients with schizophrenia in some studies (Van Mierlo and De Witte, 2018).

What theories are there about the immune system's involvement in schizophrenia?

There are several theories about the involvement of the immune system in schizophrenia, including autoimmunity, inflammation, immune system misalignment and microglia dysfunction. For example, there is a theory that autoimmunity is a mechanism that plays a role in some of the patients with schizophrenia. For example: antibodies against own receptors can disturb information processing. Another theory is that long-term mild inflammation causes cell damage and brain dysregulation. It could also be that the immune system has been "tuned" due to disturbances in development. Recent findings support the idea that microglia activated by stressful events around or after birth are associated with the loss of synapses (Van Mierlo and De Witte, 2018).

Are there any objections against these theories?

There are certainly objections. For example, many different and sometimes contradictory results are found. It may be the case that immune disorders affect only some of the patients. Immune disorders are also found in other groups of patients, for example with bipolar disorder. Thus, the immune hypothesis is certainly not specific to schizophrenia. More and better research is therefore needed.

Can you help the immune system?

A number of studies have found beneficial effects of aspirin or N-acetylcysteine. Further research is underway. In short, more research into the involvement of immune disorders in schizophrenia spectrum disorders and their treatment is needed before findings can lead to general applications (Van Mierlo and De Witte, 2018).

References

Van Mierlo Hans, De Witte Lot. 2018. "Het immuunsysteem" In Handboek schizofreniespectrumstoornissen, edited by Wiepke Cahn, Inez Myin-Germeys, Richard Bruggeman, Lieuwe de Haan. Amsterdam: De Tijdstroom.

PART 6.

OTHER PSYCHIATRIC OR PHYSICAL PROBLEMS BESIDES PSYCHOSIS

In addition to a psychosis, other psychiatric or physical problems often occur. Various studies have shown that of the patients with the classification schizophrenia approximately:

36 percent have ever suffered from social phobia;
15 percent ever meet the criteria for a panic disorder;
80 percent have ever had a major depressive disorder;
31 percent have compulsive symptoms;
14 percent have post-traumatic stress disorder;
47 percent ever meet the criteria for addiction;
15 percent have an autism spectrum disorder;
10 to 35 percent have a metabolic syndrome;
10 to 30 percent have movement disorders.

In short, there are often more problems than just psychosis. These problems can be reduced with treatment. Hence, it is worth knowing more about it.

CHAPTER 24

ANXIETY

What is anxiety?

Anxiety is a feeling or an emotion that arises because you perceive something threatening. Anxiety is normal. In fact, without anxiety or fear your chances on survival decrease. Because of anxiety you pay more attention, you do not do dangerous things and you flee when necessary. We need fear to survive. And we are not alone. All animals that can be eaten by other animals survive only by the grace of anxiety. Fear signals you to fight or flee. Because they are so important, the mechanisms that are important to anxiety or fear arose very early in evolution. Anxiety involves certain physical symptoms (palpitations, rapid breathing, nausea, sweating) and certain thoughts and behaviors (focus on what is threatening, looking for a way out, avoiding the dangerous situation). Anxiety comes in many shapes and sizes: anxiety, fear and worry.

When is anxiety not normal?

If the anxiety is greater than usual in a certain fearful situation and you get into trouble because of this, then anxiety is not normal. Or if the anxiety persists, while the threat is already over. Or if the anxiety occurs with a very small threat.

What has suspicion to do with fear and worry?

Suspicion often goes hand in hand with worry. Because you pay a lot of attention to potential danger, you overestimate risks (everything you pay attention to grows in importance). Patients often think that worrying is wise and that it helps solve problems. That is not the case: worry constantly focuses on problems, and that alone makes them grow.

It can be the same with fear. When you're scared, you pay more attention. If you pay more attention, you will see more things that might go wrong, and that will make you even more afraid.

What is a panic attack?

A panic attack is an attack of intense anxiety. About 4 percent of all people have had a panic attack in their life. We speak of a panic attack when you suddenly feel four or more of the following symptoms:

Your heart starts to beat faster.
You start to sweat.
You start to tremble.
You have the feeling that you are not getting enough air.
You start to breathe very quickly.
You feel pressure or pain in your chest.
You feel nauseous.
You are dizzy or you feel lightheaded.
You experience tingling sensations in your body.
The world looks strange or you feel separate from yourself.

Sometimes these phenomena are so frightening that you fear that you will die.

What is a Panic Disorder?

With a panic disorder you have suffered from multiple panic attacks and you are constantly afraid of having another attack. You meet the DSM 5 panic disorder classification if there are any of the following:

For at least a month after a panic attack, you are very concerned that you will get one again.

You have been very concerned about the consequences of the panic attack for at least a month. For example, you are afraid of losing your self-control, going mad, or having a heart attack. Your behavior changes. For example, you avoid certain busy places, avoid physical exertion or avoid social situations.

What can help with panic attacks?

The following tips can help when you have a panic attack:

Realize that your complaints are harmless: you are not sick, they are feelings of anxiety.

Try to breathe calmly.

Do not avoid situations that cause anxiety. If you don't leave the situation that is fearful immediately, but stay in that situation, you will find that the fear subsides on its own. It does take willpower and conviction to stay in the threatening situation for you, but if you persist long enough, the fear will subside on its own. When you flee from the fearful situation while you are still afraid, you teach yourself the wrong things, namely that your fear decreases when you flee. As a result, you will increasingly avoid the situation.

Do not consume alcohol or caffeine: these substances can increase the risk of a panic attack.

How can cognitive behavioral therapy help with panic attacks?

When you have a panic disorder, you often automatically link a physical experience (dizziness, nausea, palpitations) and a particular thought ("I'm going to pass out", "This is serious", "I'm going to die"). During cognitive therapy you try to replace these with reassuring thoughts. For example, you can tell yourself that you have never fainted during a panic attack, and therefore it is unlikely that it will happen now. You know from experience that a panic attack is nasty, but also that it is not dangerous and that the panic will disappear on its own. Sometimes suspicion is also a cause of a panic attack: if you have catastrophic thoughts about how dangerous others are, it is good to discuss this with your therapist or doctor. You can also suffer from "emotional reasoning", for example: "Because I am now anxious, there must be a threat."

It is essential in the treatment of a panic disorder that you practice "for real". The term "exposure in vivo" is used for this. This means that in real life you seek out the terrifying situation. You look for the places that you are afraid of, for example the supermarket, a square or a cinema. In those places you will practice dealing with panic. The point is that during a panic attack you stay in a fearful place until the panic disappears. That always happens. The problem, however, is that people tend to flee from panic before the anxiety diminishes. That way they teach themselves: fleeing helps, because it eases my panic. That results in the belief: avoidance is better, because then I don't have a terrible panic attack. By not escaping the fearful situation, you notice that the fear naturally subsides after a while and then you learn: I can persist and regain control.

In short, it is extremely important that you do not leave the location where the fear originated prematurely, that is, while you are still anxious. Partly for this reason, it is wise to first create a so-called fear-hierarchy: first practice in locations where you are not so scared (for example, the neighborhood supermarket) and only then go to more scary places (for example the large shopping mall in the city). It is important that you don't change the principle of 'Stay until the panic is over'. Because only then will you learn that you can overcome the fear.

What is Social Phobia [or social anxiety disorder]?

You speak of a social phobia when someone is so afraid of being in the spotlight in a group of people that someone adjusts their life accordingly. So, for example, never goes to parties or interrupts education because he has to give a presentation to a group. Most people with social phobia are afraid of criticism from people in the group. They are afraid that they are doing something ridiculous, that they will embarrass themself. Social phobia occurs in about one in ten people, and quite often in people who suffer from psychosis. The central theme is the fear of being rejected by a group of people. This fear is often linked to (self) stigma. The phobia can be the result of psychotic symptoms. Patients can hear voices that articulate the social phobic fears, for example, "Nobody likes you", "You don't belong" or "They will laugh at you." Sometimes people try to hide that they are suffering from psychosis. Then you start to pay close attention to yourself and the thought may arise that others see that you are different and that they will therefore reject you.

What helps with social anxiety disorder?

With social anxiety disorder, cognitive behavioral therapy with psychoeducation in a group can help. In a group treatment you can practice in role play and in real life with homework assignments. Critical voices are like self-critical thoughts. It can help to discuss this with others. If someone suffers from social phobia, they tend to pay particular attention to their own behavior and reactions, and especially to think about what others will think about you. You have to learn not to pay attention to yourself, but to focus your attention on others. What can help especially is learning to make mistakes and notice that it is not so bad. Many people with social phobia try to prevent mistakes at all costs, but that is precisely why they become so tense and contact is difficult. It can be very helpful to experience that a mistake (stuttering, saying something stupid, blushing) is actually just as bad as you make it yourself.

Does medication help with anxiety?

Anxiolytics, which are drugs such as oxazepam or diazepam, are often prescribed for anxiety. They also have a temporary beneficial effect. But the big problem is that you get used to it and often need more and more medication. In addition, these drugs can be addictive. That is why psychotherapy is the treatment of choice for anxiety disorders. Antidepressants can also reduce anxiety. If psychotherapy does not help [enough] and the anxiety disorder is severe, then treatment with antidepressants may be considered.

CHAPTER 25

DEPRESSION

What is the definition of a depression?

Sadness or low mood is an important characteristic of a depression, but you only speak of a depression when there is more going on. According to the DSM-5, a depressive disorder occurs when a total of five characteristics are met (during a period of at least two weeks). In addition to a low mood or loss of pleasure in almost all activities, these can include the following characteristics:

Marked weight loss without dieting;
Sleeping problems;
Move little or on the contrary be hyperactive;
Fatigue;
Feelings of worthlessness or unjustified guilt;
Reduced ability to concentrate or indecisiveness; and
Recurring thoughts of death.

Sadness on its own is an understandable response to difficulties associated with schizophrenia or other psychotic disorders and not necessarily a disorder.

How common is depression in people with schizophrenia spectrum disorder?

As is often the case, the numbers differ in different studies. About 5 to 20 percent of people with schizophrenia have major depressive disorder at the time of the study. In the population, 5 percent had a depression in the previous year. The risk of ever developing depression is about 20 percent in the healthy population. During the phase prior to a psychosis, during a psychosis and shortly after a psychosis, this percentage is much higher, namely about 60 percent. About 80 percent of people with schizophrenia spectrum disorder have had a depressive episode at some point in their lifetime.

Why is it sometimes difficult to determine whether someone with a psychosis has depression?

This may be because some depressive symptoms (such as feeling less emotions or being less energetic) resemble negative symptoms. However, in depression, someone complains of sadness or loss of pleasure, while people usually do not complain about negative symptoms. In addition, negative symptoms are often more continuous, while the severity of depressive symptoms usually varies more over time. To properly determine the severity of depressive symptoms in people with schizophrenia, a special measuring instrument has been developed, the Calgary Depression Scale for Schizophrenia.

In addition, somberness and less energy may be associated with the use of an antipsychotic in too high a dose. Too much inhibition of dopamine then results in reduced sense of meaning and loss of motivation. Also, a certain side effect called akathisia (akathisia means "inability to sit") can cause movement unrest that can be so bad that people become suicidal.

Drug, alcohol, or nicotine use can also be associated with depressed mood. Almost all people who stop taking drugs, alcohol or nicotine get a better mood in the end.

Why is it important to treat depression?

Depression sucks: you feel absolutely worthless. Depression is associated with a higher risk of suicide. In addition, depressive symptoms hinder people's recovery. Depressive symptoms are even less favorable for personal recovery than psychotic symptoms. Quality of life is most related to the severity of depressive symptoms. That is why treatment should pay attention to depression: there is a lot to be gained there.

What causes depression in people with schizophrenia spectrum disorders?

Depression can come from going through sad things, especially if you feel that there is little you can do about your situation. Depression in people with schizophrenia spectrum disorders can arise from the psychological response to a diagnosis of schizophrenia, the consequences of the condition and the stigmas of the disease. You can also feel exhausted after a difficult psychotic period. Sad feelings can also arise if too high a dose of an antipsychotic causes too much inhibition. On the other hand, well-dosed antipsychotics can also have a beneficial effect on your mood. Addiction to alcohol or cannabis, for example, can also underlie depression.

It could also be that vulnerability to schizophrenia is related to vulnerability to depression. Similar abnormalities have been found, in both people with schizophrenia and in people with depression, that indicate inflammatory or autoimmune reactions or altered activity of brain areas (Van Rooijen et al. 2018).

What effective psychotherapeutic treatments for depression are there?

Research on cognitive behavioral therapy usually focuses on the effect on psychotic symptoms, but when you put all these studies together, there is also a small to medium beneficial effect (effect size = 0.30) on the reduction of depressive symptoms. Moreover, this favorable effect was still demonstrable even after a year. Other treatments and interventions, such as social skills training and family meetings, have not been found to have a clear effect on depressive symptoms in patients with schizophrenia.

A meta-analysis of different treatments targeting physical activity showed a fairly large effect (effect size = 0.71) on depressive symptoms. This striking beneficial effect occurred when patients performed at least thirty minutes of intensive enough physical activity for at at least three times a week and maintained it for at least three months. Intensive enough means that you cannot easily keep talking during the effort.

In practice, it is sometimes very difficult for people with schizophrenia to regain physical activity. Inactivity can be related to a lack of energy or severe symptoms. But it can also be a vicious circle: because you feel tired, you move little. Because you move little, your condition decreases and you feel tired. It really pays off to get physically active. When depressed, psychoeducation, social support, and getting active will help. It can also help if you have something to do again, and can do something that you are satisfied with. And especially if you feel that others are involved with you, and that you do meaningful things (Van Rooijen et al. 2018).

Do antipsychotics help with depression?

Antipsychotics in too high a dose can cause or intensify depressive symptoms. There is some evidence that some new antipsychotics (clozapine, olanzapine, aripiprazole, amisulpride or quetiapine) have a slightly more beneficial effect than older antipsychotics or placebo on depressive symptoms in patients with schizophrenia.

Do antidepressants help patients who are already taking an antipsychotic?

There is some evidence that treatment with antidepressants in addition to antipsychotics has modest beneficial effect in patients with schizophrenia. Some antidepressants interact with antipsychotics, which can change the blood levels of the drugs or cause side effects.

Do medications like lithium or valproate help stabilize mood in depression in people with schizophrenia?

Medicines to stabilize mood in depression don't help people with schizophrenia. Meta-analyzes show no beneficial effect on mood.

Does electroconvulsive therapy help with depression in patients with schizophrenia?

Electroconvulsive therapy (ECT) can help with persisting psychosis, even when patients are treated with clozapine. Since ECT is helpful for people with depression that is not improving, you would expect ECT to also help people with schizophrenia who remain depressed. But research has not found any indications for this.

Does repetitive transcranial magnetic stimulation help with depression in patients with schizophrenia?

Repetitive transcranial magnetic stimulation (rTMS) can reduce hearing voices or negative symptoms, but there is no clear evidence yet that rTMS has a beneficial effect on depression in schizophrenia.

What does the step-by-step plan for the treatment of depressive symptoms in someone with schizophrenia look like?

If someone in the acute phase of a psychosis suffers from additional depression, it is best to start treatment with an antipsychotic. It is important that the dose is not too high and there is some preference for clozapine, olanzapine, aripiprazole, amisulpride or quetiapine.

If the symptoms of depression persist, the next treatment step is to increase physical activities. According to research, if someone performs physical activities of a considerable intensity for at least thirty minutes for at least three times a week, and maintains this for at least three months, this has a beneficial effect.

Scientific research does not provide clear indications for the next step. Whether this is psychotherapy or treatment with an antidepressant depends on patient preference and availability (Van Rooijen et al. 2018).

References

Van Rooijen Geeske, Ruhe Eric, De Haan Lieuwe. 2018. "Depressieve stoornis" In Handboek schizofreniespectrumstoornissen, edited by Wiepke Cahn, Inez Myin-Germeys, Richard Bruggeman, Lieuwe de Haan. Amsterdam: De Tijdstroom.

CHAPTER 26

TRAUMA

What is Psychotrauma?

Psychotrauma (also: psychological trauma) is psychological injury that someone suffers after a horrible event.

What kind of trauma can you suffer during a psychosis?

Sometimes patients experience unpleasant things during their psychosis. Admission to a psychiatric ward, a stay in an isolation room or forced administration of medication can be very traumatizing.

What kind trauma can arise after a psychosis?

Sometimes people get trauma after the psychotic period has passed. People who become homeless or addicted in particular run a high risk of being robbed, and the chance of experiencing sexual violence is also higher.

What kind of trauma can occur prior to psychosis?

Child maltreatment and sexual abuse occur in patients who later develop psychotic complaints. In particular, repeated sexual abuse in youth increases the chance of developing psychosis in adulthood. Based on findings in a meta-analysis, it is assumed that trauma can be a direct cause of psychosis. And the authors estimate that even one third of new cases of psychotic illness may be explained by serious trauma. Hallucinations can refer to the trauma or to keeping it secret (Van de Berg and Van der Gaag 2018).

What is Post Traumatic Stress Disorder?

People with post-traumatic stress disorder suffer from three types of symptoms: re-experiencing, avoidance, and tension. Below I describe these symptoms in more detail.

The main phenomenon of post-traumatic stress disorder is re-experiencing. During re-experiencing it seems as if you are experiencing the traumatic event again. Without you wanting to, unpleasant memories of the trauma come back to you. You can also have nightmares about the trauma. Those memories or nightmares can be very realistic and make you very anxious. Because everything that reminds you of the trauma is so bad, you try to avoid things related to the trauma. This can go so far that you shut yourself off from contact with all people, and that your feelings flatten. You are also more irritable and tense than before the trauma. This can manifest itself in difficulty falling asleep or sleeping through, irritability, outbursts of anger or excessive alertness and vigilance. In one year, about 3.5 percent of the population suffers from post-traumatic stress disorder.

Why is it that one person develops post-traumatic stress disorder after a traumatic event and the other does not?

We do not know why after a traumatic event one develops a post-traumatic stress disorder and the other does not. We do know a number of factors that increase the risk of post-traumatic stress disorder. Wars and sex crimes cause post-traumatic stress disorders more often than natural disasters: the most traumatic is what people do to each other. The more often shocking events occur, the more difficult they are to process. Some people are more sensitive than others. If you have experienced little support from others earlier and after the trauma, you have a higher risk to suffer from a post traumatic stress disorder is larger.

How often do people with psychosis suffer from post-traumatic stress disorder?

Of the patients with a psychotic disorder, 12 to 16 percent also meet the criteria for a post-traumatic stress disorder. Trauma in childhood is common in the population and is associated with psychiatric problems in adulthood. A review article found that about 50 percent of women with psychosis and about 20 percent of men with psychosis had experienced childhood sexual abuse. Other traumatic experiences, such as abuse and neglect, are also relatively common in people with a psychotic illness. In addition, people with psychosis are also more likely to experience traumatic experiences during their psychosis and in the time afterwards (Van de Berg and Van der Gaag 2018).

Are the symptoms of people who have both a psychosis and a post-traumatic stress disorder different from those of people who "only" suffer from a psychosis?

People with psychosis who also suffer from a post-traumatic stress disorder have more serious complaints, function less well and have a lower quality of life than people who "alone" suffer from a psychosis. They also use more antipsychotics, to which they respond less well on average. Moreover, collaboration with professional caregiver is often more difficult (Van de Berg and Van der Gaag 2018).

How can trauma affect the nature of psychotic symptoms?

Hallucinations can sometimes be directly related to the trauma, such as when voices berate you in the same way as when you were sexually assaulted. Your beliefs may also have been shaped by the trauma, for example, the belief that you are not worth it because it is all your own fault. Core beliefs about yourself, others, and the world, also called cognitive schemas, can play an important role in delusions. For example, a negative self-image coupled with a hostile image of the other increases the chance of developing paranoid delusions. Your core beliefs are influenced by what you experience and by your contact with the people who took care of you or should have done so. These core beliefs influence how you interpret situations. For example, someone who distrusts others and feels vulnerable is more prone to suspicion

What is the treatment for people who have post-traumatic stress disorder?

There are two effective forms of trauma treatment for post-traumatic stress disorder: Eye Movement Desensitization and Reprocessing (EMDR) and Prolonged Exposure (PE). I discuss them in more detail below.

How does EMDR work?

During an EMDR treatment you go back to the shocking event in your mind. You reflect on what you feel, what you see and what your thoughts are about the traumatic event. Ultimately, you focus on the most dire memory of the trauma. While you do this, the EMDR therapist is distracting you. For example, by making a finger movement that you have to follow with your eyes or by making alternating beeps heard through headphones. By repeatedly reflecting on the memory you are afraid of and being distracted at the same time, the emotional memory is processed less well. It is thought that memories are then re-stored, but in a less emotionally charged form. That would be because the capacity of the working memory is limited: you cannot properly register two things at the same time. After the treatment, it may become easier to think about the traumatic event. In this way the trauma can take on a less threatening meaning. Complaints such as intrusive memories, fearful images, re-experiences, flashbacks and nightmares can then disappear or greatly diminish (Van de Berg and Van der Gaag 2018).

How does Prolonged Exposure work?

There is some evidence that direct exposure to traumatic memories is most effective. In order to achieve this, it appears that the emotional intensity must be high enough during the treatment. PE is based on the idea that prolonged exposure to anxious feelings and thoughts ultimately results in a decrease in re-experiencing, avoidance and tension. During the treatment you will be asked to talk about the traumatic event as if you were reliving the trauma. You are stimulated to dwell in detail on the most painful and fearful moments. So, you confront yourself intensively and for a relatively long time with the traumatic event. At the beginning of the treatment, anxiety often increases, but after that, habituation occurs. Probably, it plays a role that emotional re-experience strengthens self-confidence: I can handle this nasty memory and will not lose it.

Recently it was found that also less intensive therapies may improve post-traumatic stress disorder. Six sessions of 30 minutes of writing about the trauma resulted in comparable improvement as prolonged exposure (Van de Berg and Van der Gaag 2018).

What is the problem in the treatment of people who have psychosis and post-traumatic stress disorder?

Post-traumatic stress disorder is usually not recognized in people with a psychotic illness. Very often, post-traumatic stress disorder is not treated because clinicians are afraid that treatment will cause a person with psychosis to become more unbalanced. Patients also often do not dare to take such a treatment, and therapists do not want to insist or do not dare to do so. Psychosis is usually a reason for not allowing people to participate in research into the effectiveness of trauma-focused therapy. The research that has been carried out with people with psychosis shows that trauma therapy does not cause people to become unbalanced more often or more seriously. On the contrary, there is more balance and less crisis in people with psychosis and post-traumatic stress disorder who receive trauma treatment. So, while both trauma and post-traumatic stress disorder are very common in people with psychosis, they are both often missed and often left untreated (Van de Berg and Van der Gaag 2018).

How effective is trauma-focused therapy in psychosis?

In some non-blinded studies without a control group, a large beneficial effect of six sessions of EMDR or PE was found. Following this favorable evidence, trauma-focused therapy was investigated in 155 participants with chronic post-traumatic stress disorder and psychosis in a randomized controlled trial. Before PE or EMDR was applied, no psychotherapy aimed at increasing the stability of people took place. In about 60 percent of the treated participants, the complaints no longer met the criteria of a post-traumatic stress disorder after the treatment. In the group on the waiting list, there was no improvement noticeable. Crisis occurred less often in the group of people receiving treatment. Also, negative and positive symptoms decreased in severity in the group receiving trauma treatment (Van de Berg and Van der Gaag 2018).

Why is an intervention aimed at stabilization not necessary befor trauma treatment?

There are no indications that an intervention aimed at stabilization is necessary for trauma treatment in patients with a psychosis. With stabilization treatment, therapists could inadvertently send out the message that the trauma treatment is dangerous for the patient, that they may not be able to cope with the treatment, that they are too difficult a case to treat, or that they themselves find it exciting to have the treatment at the patient. This could make patients more anxious and give less hope for a good outcome (Van de Berg and Van der Gaag 2018).

What could explain the beneficial effects of trauma treatment on other symptoms?

This could perhaps be explained by network theory. Network theory assumes that symptoms influence each other. In this case, central or dominant symptoms could influence several other symptoms. It may be that symptoms of post-traumatic stress play a central role, and that if these central symptoms decrease, other symptoms also improve.

References

Van de Berg David, Van der Gaag Mark. 2018. “Post traumatische stress stoornis” In Handboek schizofreniespectrumstoornissen, edited by Wiepke Cahn, Inez Myin-Germeys, Richard Bruggeman, Lieuwe de Haan. Amsterdam: De Tijdstroom.

CHAPTER 27

ADDICTION

What are the criteria for the classification addiction?

We speak of an addiction when the use of cannabis, nicotine, alcohol or other drugs leads to problems. The DSM-5 lists eleven characteristics, two of which you must have, to meet the classification "substance use disorder".

In this chapter, I refer to this classification by the term "addiction."

Following are the eleven DSM-5 characteristics of an addiction:

1 use more or longer drugs than intended;
2 persistent desire or unsuccessful attempts to use less substances;
3 spend a lot of time obtaining and using the substance, or recovering from use;
4 cravings for substances;
5 repeated use causing problems at school, work or at home;
6 continue to use despite recurring social problems caused by the drug;
7 spend less time on social activities, work, or hobbies;
8 repeated occurrence of danger caused by substance use;
9 continuing substance use despite the presence of a physical or psychological problem caused or aggravated by the use;
10 Use more to get the desired effect (habituation);
11 withdrawal symptoms.

If you meet two or three of the criteria, it is considered a mild addiction. If you meet four or five of the criteria, you have a moderately severe addiction. If you meet six or more criteria, you are dealing with a serious addiction.

Why is addiction more common in people with a schizophrenia spectrum disorder?

There are several theories as to why addiction is more common in people with schizophrenia spectrum disorder. Substance use could be a causal or triggering factor of a psychotic illness. In the first case - if it were a decisive causal factor - the schizophrenia spectrum disorder would not have developed without the presence of substance use. In the second case: if substance use is a triggering factor, the disorder would probably have developed even without the substance use, but later or only under less favorable circumstances. Another theory is that having schizophrenia spectrum disorder leads to substance use and, ultimately, addiction. This could be because patients with schizophrenia spectrum disorders try to reduce symptoms of their disease or side effects of antipsychotics with the help of addictive substances. For example, patients would try to improve their condition with drugs, but would end up worse. They may sometimes feel better, but they develop an addiction. A third possible explanation for the co-occurrence of schizophrenia and addiction is the presence of common risk factors. Finally, it could also be the case that one problem adversely affects the course of the other.

Is drug use increasing worldwide?

round 284 million people aged 15-64 used drugs worldwide in 2020. This is about a 25% increase over the previous decade. Young people are using more drugs. The majority of people treated for drug disorders are under 35.

In the paragraphs below, I will discuss the individual addictive substances separately. Then I will also discuss what we know about the cause of addiction.

Cannabis

How common is cannabis use in the population?

Cannabis has been one of the most commonly used types of drugs in the Western world for years. In Israel about 27% of the adult population used cannabis at least once in 2020. In the United States this figure is about 17%. In the United Kingdom this figure is about 7%. About 25 percent of current cannabis users use the drug on a daily basis and nearly half of this group develops cannabis addiction. In the United States, sales of legal cannabis are expected to reach an estimated 37 billion U.S. dollars by 2026. Cannabis legalization in parts of the world may have accelerated daily use. The percentages of current cannabis use are higher in groups of young people with problems: 45 percent among young people in youth care, 55 percent among young people who drop out of school prematurely and 87 percent among young homeless people.

How common is cannabis use in patients with schizophrenia?

In a recent Dutch study, 80 percent of patients with schizophrenia were found to have ever used cannabis, while at least 35 percent of patients were still found to use cannabis regularly when admitted to a psychiatric hospital. This percentage is higher in patients who are admitted with a first psychosis: up to about 60 percent.

What is the relationship between cannabis use and schizophrenia?

We know from research that cannabis use is clearly associated with the risk of developing psychotic symptoms and schizophrenia spectrum disorders. In addition, the risk of a psychotic disorder increases if someone smokes a lot and / or starts smoking young and / or uses THC-rich cannabis. This association between cannabis use and schizophrenia spectrum disorders could be caused by another factors. For example, young people with problems smoke often, and not so much the smoking as the fact that they have many problems is associated with the risk of a psychotic disorder. But even if you combine the results of all the studies and take these underlying factors into account, the risk of a psychotic illness is still more than twice as high when someone often uses cannabis. About 10 percent of all new schizophrenia cases could be attributed to cannabis use, assuming that the cannabis use is 100 percent causal.

Research has also found that some smokers are more at risk of developing a psychotic illness than others. The highest risk applies to young people who start smoking before the age of 15 and to people who have someone with a psychotic disorder in their family.

Recent research shows that genes associated with an increased risk of schizophrenia are also associated with a greater risk that someone will use (a lot of) cannabis. The biological vulnerability of the cannabinoid or glutamatergic system is thought to contribute to both schizophrenia and cannabis addiction. Furthermore, adverse factors in early childhood, such as neglect or abuse, can also influence the risk of both schizophrenia and cannabis addiction.

Why do patients use cannabis?

Patients with schizophrenia spectrum disorders say they use cannabis for relaxation and socializing, but also because they then suffer less from depression, fear, restlessness or boredom. In addition, they expect and experience that cannabis use makes social contact easier. Yet other research shows that cannabis use is also a risk factor for the development of depressive symptoms and anxiety, and it has also been shown that when patients stop smoking, their mood and motivation improve. About half of the patients with schizophrenia spectrum disorders who are advised to discontinue, do so.

What is the influence of cannabis use on the course of schizophrenia spectrum disorders?

Cannabis use, and certainly cannabis addiction, adversely affect the course of schizophrenia spectrum disorders. Blowers are more likely to have severe psychosis, have more psychotic episodes, show more aggression, function less socially, are more often admitted to psychiatric institutions and have more judicial contacts.

On the other hand, the cognitive functioning of the group of patients who have used cannabis in the past is better than that of patients who have never used cannabis. This is discussed in more detail in the next section.

How is it possible that former smokers have better information processing capacities (provided they are not stoned)?

The explanation for this could be that people who develop schizophrenia after using cannabis for a period of time "needed" this extra risk factor to actually experience psychosis. People who become psychotic without ever smoking cannabis are probably extra vulnerable to develop psychosis or schizophrenia, which can also manifest itself in less good cognitive functioning. Cognitive functioning is clearly worse if someone is under the influence of cannabis at the time of the test. In other words, the former users themselves had less problems processing information and the use of cannabis gave them the necessary push to develop a psychosis. Patients who have never used cannabis have not needed this additional risk factor to develop schizophrenia. In other words: they were naturally more vulnerable, and this is also reflected in their limited ability to process information. It is indisputable that stopping using cannabis is beneficial for the development of patients with schizophrenia spectrum disorders. And it is also perfectly clear that not being stoned is good for the quality of your information processing.

Nicotine

How many people smoke worldwide?

In 2020, 22.3% of the world's population used tobacco: 36.7% of men and 7.8% of women. Nicotine use remains high in particular among adolescents [about 30%]. Tobacco kills up to half of its users. Tobacco kills more than 8 million people each year, including 1.3 million non-smokers who are exposed to second-hand smoke.

How often do patients with schizophrenia smoke?

About 80 percent of people with schizophrenia smoke. In addition, they are more likely to be a heavy smoker (25 cigarettes or more per day). Smoking is therefore the leading cause of premature death in people with schizophrenia. This makes cutting back on smoking a top priority.

Why is it that patients with schizophrenia spectrum disorders smoke so much?

It was sometimes thought that patients smoke to improve their cognitive function. However, the most recent overview study shows that there is no evidence to support the proposition that nicotine has a beneficial effect on the cognitive functioning of patients with schizophrenia. Moreover, a recent study showed that quitting smoking in patients with schizophrenia is associated with an improvement in the speed of information processing. The more patients smoked, the worse their information processing speed and problem solving abilities. Smoking may be related to a higher dose of antipsychotic medication. It was found that patients of whom a higher percentage of their dopamine D_2 receptors were occupied by antipsychotics tended to smoke much more cigarettes. Probably this is related to the reduction in blood level of antipsychotics caused by smoking cigarettes. Probably patients try to lower a too high blood level of antipsychotics through smoking.

Once you start smoking, it can be very difficult to give up permanently. Smoking is extremely addictive. Every cigarette gives an addictive flash of nicotine, which makes you momentarily feel better. That is why it is important that as few people as possible start smoking and that people receive intensive help to stop. Quitting smoking gives a lot of health benefits. Hardly any other therapeutic intervention can compete with this.

Alcohol

How much alcohol is consumed worldwide?

Total alcohol consumption per year in 2016 was on average 19.4 litres of pure alcohol for males and 7.0 litres for females.

What are the somatic health consequences of alcohol use?

The harmful use of alcohol is a causal factor in more than 200 diseases and injuries. Worldwide, 3 million deaths every year result from harmful use of alcohol. This represents 5.3% of all deaths. Alcohol consumption causes death and disability relatively early in life. In people aged 20–39 years, approximately 14% of total deaths are attributable to alcohol.

How many people with schizophrenia have ever been addicted to alcohol?

About 20 percent of people with schizophrenia have ever been addicted to alcohol. About 40 percent of people with schizophrenia and alcohol addiction have another addiction, usually nicotine.

Is there a relationship between alcohol consumption and schizophrenia?

Although alcohol addiction and schizophrenia often occur together, there is no evidence that alcohol consumption contributes to the development of schizophrenia. There are also no indications that the same genes play a role in the development of both schizophrenia and alcohol abuse.

What reasons do people with schizophrenia give for their alcohol consumption?

Fighting sadness and anxiety is often cited as a motivation for alcohol use by patients with schizophrenia, but it could also be the other way around that sadness arises from excessive alcohol consumption. It is clear that cognitive functioning is worse if people with schizophrenia are addicted to alcohol. In addition, aggressive behavior is more common in patients with schizophrenia and alcohol addiction. When people stop drinking, their mood improves and they feel better.

Cocaine

How many people use cocaine worldwide?

In 2020 there were about 22 million people using cocaine. That group consists of about three times more men than women.

How many people with schizophrenia have ever used cocaine?

It is estimated that about 30 percent of individuals with schizophrenia have ever used cocaine.

Can cocaine use lead to schizophrenia?

It is clear that cocaine use can cause (paranoid) delusions and / or hallucinations, even in people who are not very vulnerable to developing schizophrenia. Usually, psychotic symptoms disappear when people stop using cocaine. Cocaine use is probably associated with a greater risk of developing schizophrenia. The risk of developing a new psychosis is substantially larger if someone with an increased vulnerability to schizophrenia uses cocaine. Furthermore, of all addictive substances, cocaine appears to be most strongly associated with an exacerbation of motor side effects with antipsychotics.

Treatment of patients with schizophrenia and addiction

Are certain antipsychotics better or worse in addicted patients?

Too few good studies have been done to provide indisputable recommendations for the use of antipsychotics in patients with addiction. Nevertheless, there are many indications that, in addition to beneficial effects on psychotic symptoms, clozapine reduces the severity of addiction. Furthermore, there is some evidence that people who receive relatively high doses of an antipsychotic drug that attaches vigorously to the dopamine receptor (e.g. haloperidol or risperidone) are more likely to smoke and have more cannabis craving.

Are there safe and effective drugs for alcohol addiction in patients with psychosis?

Naltrexone and disulfiram are safe and effective medications to treat alcohol dependence in patients with schizophrenia.

Is there an appropriate pharmacological treatment of cannabis dependence in patients with schizophrenia?

There is no suitable pharmacological treatment of cannabis dependence in patients with schizophrenia. Recently, an attempt to replace "street cannabis" with a CBD-rich and low-THC form failed because this low-THC cannabis was not appreciated by patients and they started using street cannabis again.

What are the drug treatment options for patients with schizophrenia and tobacco addiction?

Varenicline or bupropion are effective for tobacco addiction. Nicotine replacement therapies, for example nicotine patches, are also effective when prescribed for more than six months. The combination treatment of nicotine replacement and bupropion increases the effectiveness.

Will you get depressed when you quit smoking?

When you quit smoking, you have to get used to the disappearance of the effect of nicotine. It is therefore recommended to use nicotine replacement when attempting to quit and to maintain treatment with nicotine tablets, patches or gum for a long time, i.e. longer than six months. No increase in depression was seen in the group thus treated. In fact, your quality of life improves and your mood improves after stopping smoking.

Which psychotherapeutic addiction treatments are effective?

A large meta-analysis does not reveal any indications that one form of psychotherapy for addiction is better than another. Motivational and cognitive-behavioral therapies have been found to be most effective in patients (see also Chapter 42 on psychotherapy). A special form of therapy, namely training for parents in interactive and motivational skills, was also found to be effective in reducing cannabis use in young people with schizophrenia.

What principles can help reduce the severity of addiction?

The following "principles" can help reduce the severity of addiction:

First, go for damage control instead of stopping completely. The treatment of addiction in psychosis is more successful if the goal is to limit damage than if the goal is to stop using addictive substances altogether.

Second, avoid places where addictive substances are used and look for other things that you enjoy.

Third, don't be put off by a slip. A relapse in use is not a sign that you have lost it all, but means that you can start decreasing again tomorrow. Moreover, you can learn from a slip.

Fourth, practice saying no.

Fifth, identify the pros and cons of using addictive substances.

Finally, it may seem that substance use helps you bear the consequences of your condition, but research shows that the quality of life actually improves when you manage to quit. No matter how difficult that may be in the beginning.

CHAPTER 28

OBSESSIONS AND COMPULSIONS

What are obsessions?

Compulsive thoughts are recurring or persistent thoughts that you experience as misplaced and burdensome. People who have obsessive thoughts know that these thoughts are exaggerated and that they produce the thoughts themselves, but they cannot stop or ignore them.

What are compulsions?

Compulsions are repetitive behaviors - such as washing hands, checking a lock, or performing rituals - that a person feels compelled to do, often in response to obsessions. The purpose of the compulsions is to prevent disaster. These behaviors do not show a realistic relationship with the event to be neutralized. People realize that the compulsions are exaggerated or unjustified. Yet they can hardly, if at all, stop or reduce the actions.

What is an Obsessive Compulsive Disorder?

When people are often disturbed by obsessive thoughts and actions and they spend more than an hour a day on them, we call it an obsessive-compulsive disorder.

Do obsessive compulsive symptoms occur in healthy people?

Milder compulsive thoughts or actions are common. About 20 percent of the population sometimes suffers from this.

A common and mild compulsion is to check repeatedly whether you have locked the door when you go on holyday. You actually know you've locked the door, but you're not quite sure. And you want to be. After all, you are leaving for a long time. You are not comfortable. You are already on your way to the train and yet you decide to turn around, to check once more whether you have really closed the door properly.

How can you distinguish obsessions from delusions?

Delusions and obsessions are similar in a number of ways, but there are also differences. An obsession is an unwanted, persistent thought that the person recognizes as being nonsensical or irrational but nevertheless originates out of his own thoughts. A delusion is also often irrational, but you experience this belief as realistic. Understanding the irrational nature of an obsession and resisting against an obsession are the most important distinctions from a delusion. Compulsive thoughts and actions are characterized by gnawing insecurity, while delusions involve an unshakable conviction. In terms of content, there is often also a difference between delusions and obsessions. Delusions often involve suspicion, ideas of reference, a sense of grandeur or spirituality, while obsessions and compulsions often involve fear of contamination, sexual themes or averting disaster, or order or control (De Haan et al. 2018).

How common are obsessions and compulsions in patients with schizophrenia?

A meta-analysis showed that more than 30 percent of patients with schizophrenia occasionally suffer from obsessive thoughts or actions. In 12 percent of the patients, these complaints were so bad that they met the DSM criteria for obsessive-compulsive disorder. This is far more substantial than in the general population: obsessive-compulsive disorder occurs in about 1 percent of people. As mentioned earlier, about 20 percent of the population has occasionally suffered from obsessive thoughts or acts (De Haan et al. 2018).

Are the causes of obsessions/compulsive and psychosis related?

There are a number of indications for a connection between the causes of compulsive complaints and psychosis. People with obsessive-compulsive disorder are 12 times more likely to have schizophrenia and people with schizophrenia are 12 times more likely to have obsessive-compulsive disorder. First, second and third degree family members also share the risk of both conditions. In addition, a common factor has also been found that can increase vulnerability to both conditions: people who have experienced a toxoplasmosis infection are almost twice as likely to develop schizophrenia and more than three times as likely to develop an obsessive-compulsive disorder. Therefore, obsessive compulsive disorders and psychosis have probably common causes or risk factors (De Haan et al. 2018).

What is the course of obsessions/compulsions in people with schizophrenia?

In about 50 percent of people with schizophrenia who also suffer from obsessions/compulsions, these symptoms develop before psychotic symptoms occur. In another group, psychotic symptoms and obsessions/compulsions arise and disappear simultaneously. Finally, there is a group of patients whose obsessions/compulsions develop after the onset of the psychosis. In that case, the compulsive symptoms are sometimes related to the use of clozapine. In most patients, the severity of the discomfort they experience from obsessive symptoms varies. About 12 percent of patients with schizophrenia have long-term obsessions/compulsions. These patients often require adjustment of treatment (De Haan et al. 2018).

Are obsessions/compulsions related to other symptoms?

People with schizophrenia who suffer from obsessions/compulsions for a longer period of time are often more depressed and function less well. People with persistent obsessions/compulsions are also more likely to be overly concerned and less confident in their own ability to solve problems. That is why it is important to treat persistent obsessions/compulsions.

Do antipsychotics affect obsessions/compulsions?

Obsessions/compulsions are more common in people who use clozapine for a long time. Research shows that this occurs in about 30 percent of patients taking clozapine. For some this is a serious problem. Pre-existing obsessions/compulsions worsen in about 15 percent of patients. To make matters even more complicated, obsessions/compulsions actually improve in about 10 percent of patients treated with clozapine (De Haan et al. 2018).

What is the drug treatment of choice for permanent severe obsessions/compulsions in someone with schizophrenia?

The primary consideration in the case of persistent severe obsessions/compulsions in someone with schizophrenia, should be whether the obsessions/compulsions develop or have worsened after starting treatment with antipsychotics. If so, consideration may be given to dose reduction or a switch to an antipsychotic with a more favorable side effect profile, such as aripiprazole. In addition, a study showed that olanzapine had a more beneficial effect on the severity of obsessions/compulsions than risperidone.

If a dose reduction or switch to another antipsychotic is not desirable, the addition of an antidepressant may have beneficial effects on obsessions/ compulsions. 150 milligrams of fluvoxamine per day is the best-studied antidepressant in these cases. Antidepressants can affect the enzymes that break down drugs. Certainly, with clozapine, the blood level must therefore be closely monitored. The dosage of antipsychotics should be adjusted when antidepressants and antipsychotics are used concomitantly (De Haan et al. 2018).

What is the psychotherapeutic treatment of permanent severe obsessions/compulsions in someone with schizophrenia?

Cognitive behavioral therapy helps people with 'only' obsessions/ compulsions and also people with schizophrenia and obsessions/ compulsions. Little research has been conducted into the effect of cognitive behavioral therapy on obsessions/compulsions in schizophrenia, but the available results are encouraging. Cognitive behavioral therapy had a beneficial effect in about 80 percent of the patients, but that high percentage was found in studies without a control group. The beneficial effect of cognitive behavioral therapy on obsessions/compulsions in people with schizophrenia has therefore not been proven.

References

De Haan Lieuwe, Swets Marije, Schoevers Robert. 2018. "Obessieve-compulsieve stoornis" In Handboek schizofreniespectrumstoornissen, edited by Wiepke Cahn, Inez Myin-Germeys, Richard Bruggeman, Lieuwe de Haan. Amsterdam: De Tijdstroom.

CHAPTER 29

MENTAL DISABILITY

When do you speak of a very mild intellectual disability?

People with an IQ between 70 and 85 meet the classification 'very mildly mentally disabled'. People with a very mild intellectual disability often have difficulties in communication, self-care, living independently, social skills and making independent decisions. They generally have a developmental age of about twelve to thirteen years. At that age, the development of personal responsibility and conscience has not been completed.

When do you speak of a mild intellectual disability?

People with an IQ between 50 and 70 are said to be mildly mentally disabled. About 10 to 15 percent of the population has an IQ between 50 and 85. Someone with a mild intellectual disability has about the cognitive developmental level of a six to eleven year old. The emotional development of people with a mild intellectual disability often reaches the so-called identification phase. In the identification phase you need another identification figure, that is to say: your self-image is not yet developed to the extent that you can "stand on your own". It is also often difficult to distinguish between reality and fantasy in this phase.

Is a (very) mild intellectual disability more common in people with a schizophrenia spectrum disorder?

Schizophrenia is slightly more common in very smart people and more often occurs in people who are less than average intelligent. Therefore, it is roughly estimated that about 20 percent of people with schizophrenia spectrum disorder have an IQ between 50 and 85.

What should the professional caregiver take into account in the treatment of someone with a psychosis and a (very) mild intellectual disability?

In the treatment of someone with a psychosis and a (very) mild intellectual disability, an explanation about the condition and the treatment must be simple in the first place, so that it can be understood by the patient. The information in this book is generally difficult to understand for someone with mild intellectual disabilities. Second, it must be taken into account that some problems may be related to a person's level of development. Suppose someone finds it difficult to be alone. This may have to do with the level of development. For example, someone with an IQ of 60 has the developmental level of a toddler, and it is quite normal for toddlers to not tolerate being alone well. Problems arise if the environment is insufficiently attuned to a patient's cognitive, social and emotional skills. Others must also take into account that people with a (very) mild intellectual disability may have a reduced sense of time and also have a reduced ability to distinguish between fantasy and reality. In addition, awareness of the relationship between cause and effect may be limited.

In people with a (very) mild intellectual disability, the environment has even more influence on the development and persistence of psychological complaints than in people without an intellectual disability. That is why it is important to find out which environmental influences are beneficial and which are unfavorable.

Sometimes a (very) mild intellectual disability is also related to a certain genetic abnormality. If there are indications that this may be the case, it may be wise to do genetic consultation.

Finally, it is important to be aware of drug side effects and paradoxical reactions, meaning that with medication, the opposite effect of what was intended is achieved (for example, someone on a sedative gets very upset). Side effects and paradoxical reactions are more common in people with a (very) mild intellectual disability.

CHAPTER 30

AUTISM

What is Autism Spectrum Disorder?

Autism spectrum disorder is a developmental disorder that manifests itself in childhood, with limitations in the reciprocity of social contacts and communication, and with limited and little changeable interests and behaviors.

The DSM-5 classification system describes the following criteria for an autism spectrum disorder:

1. There must be persistent deficits in social communication and social interaction, as shown by:
   a. Deficits in social-emotional reciprocity (for example: abnormal social approach, difficulty with conversations); and
   b. Deficiencies in non-verbal communication (e.g. difficulty with eye contact, difficulty with understanding and using gestures); and
   c. Deficits in developing, maintaining, and understanding relationships (e.g., difficulty adapting behavior to the environment, difficulty making friends, or little interest in peers).
2. There must be limited, repetitive patterns of behavior, interests, or activities, as evidenced by:
   a. Repeated movements or repeated use of objects or speech;
   b. Sticking to routines, difficulty with change;
   c. Very limited, unchanging interests;
   d. Sensory hypersensitivity or insensitivity.

To meet the DSM-5 autism spectrum disorder classification, the above symptoms must be present from an early age.

Are psychotic symptoms more common in people with autism spectrum disorder?

Some studies show that delusions and / or hallucinations occur in about a third of people with autism spectrum disorder. On the other hand, there are also studies that show no evidence of an increased incidence of psychosis in people with an autism spectrum disorder. If the delusions and / or hallucinations cause long-term discomfort and if the other criteria of schizophrenia are also met, then this classification is placed next to the autism spectrum disorder.

Both autism spectrum disorder and schizophrenia affect about 1 percent of the population. A meta-analysis shows that about 13 percent of people with autism spectrum disorder also meet the criteria for schizophrenia and that about 4 percent of people with schizophrenia can also be classified as having an autism spectrum disorder.

Do abnormalities in social cognition occur in both schizophrenia and autism spectrum disorder?

Social cognition concerns the processing of social information. Examples are recognizing emotions in facial expressions or being able to empathize with the other. Less good social cognition is a core phenomenon of the autism spectrum disorder, but this can also occur in schizophrenia.

What do we know about the genetics of autism spectrum disorder and schizophrenia?

Genetic vulnerability plays a major role in both schizophrenia and autism spectrum disorder. Variation in copying errors (so-called Copy Number Variation) occurs in both schizophrenia and autism spectrum disorder. However, studies of common genetic variation show that schizophrenia and autism spectrum disorder differ from each other. Genome-wide association studies found only a correlation of 0.16 between autism spectrum disorder and schizophrenia. For example, the correlation between bipolar disorder and schizophrenia was much larger: 0.68.

What can be said in general about neurobiological research into autism spectrum disorder and schizophrenia?

In schizophrenia a decrease in total brain volume is found, while in autism spectrum disorder showed an increase in total brain volume is found. A less rigid organization of the white matter bundles has been found in both disorders. A meta-analysis found decreased activity in brain areas related to social cognition in both schizophrenia and autism spectrum disorder. On the other hand, there are also studies that found an increased activity in schizophrenia and a reduced activity of these areas in autism spectrum disorder.

Electroencephalography research can estimate the activity of mirror neurons that are important for social behavior. In schizophrenia, indications were found of increased activity, while in autism spectrum disorder there were indications of decreased activity.

In both schizophrenia and autism spectrum disorder, indications have been found of increased activity in the dopamine system in the basal nuclei. Evidence of subtle inflammation in the brain is found in both conditions. Whether there are differences between the two disorders in terms of inflammation is not yet clear.

The neurological research thus shows both overlap and difference between autism spectrum disorder and schizophrenia. Whether there is a shared vulnerability or whether there are certain subtypes within these two disorders where the overlap is greater than with other subtypes is not yet clear (Maat and Palmen 2018).

What could be the consequences of difficulties in distinguishing between autism spectrum disorder and schizophrenia?

Specila ideas held by someone with an autism spectrum disorder may resemble delusions in schizophrenia. It could then be wrongly treated with antipsychotic medication. Because patients with autism spectrum disorder may be more sensitive to the side effects of antipsychotics, this could have additional adverse effects. On the other hand, withdrawal behavior and suspicious thoughts in someone with schizophrenia can sometimes be interpreted as signs of an autism spectrum disorder. This can lead to no antipsychotics being prescribed, while that could actually improve the condition.

What do some researchers think about the relationship between schizophrenia and autism spectrum disorder?

Some researchers view both schizophrenia and the autism spectrum disorder as neurodevelopmental disorders. These conditions can co-occur. These researchers argue for a dimensional approach, in which they draw attention to certain characteristics of schizophrenia or the autism spectrum disorder that may be present to a greater or lesser extent.

Which interventions can help in case of autism spectrum disorder?

There are no drugs that help with autism spectrum disorder. However, it can help to take more account of the limitations (and qualities!) of people with this disorder. Interventions that focus on coping with cognitive skills and mutual adaptations of behavior and environment can help. This does not remove the core problems of autism, but the anxiety and fear can diminish. Moreover, this can improve contact between parents and children with autism. General principles that have beneficial effects are clarity and structure.

Sometimes antidepressants are used in case of the occurrence of repetitive thoughts or behavior. These drugs may reduce irritability. Sometimes antipsychotics are given to reduce aggressive behavior. Both drugs are then prescribed off-label: that is, there is no good research on which to base this application (Maat and Palmen 2018).

Which factors need attention in the treatment of people who suffer from psychosis or schizophrenia and who also have an autism spectrum disorder?

Hardly any research has been conducted into the pharmacological or psychotherapeutic treatment of people who suffer from the combination of psychosis or schizophrenia and an autism spectrum disorder. However, there is some evidence that people with autism spectrum disorder are more sensitive to motor and metabolic side effects of antipsychotics. Furthermore, experience shows that patients with an autism spectrum disorder feel less at ease in a group and could therefore benefit more from individual therapy (Maat and Palmen 2018).

References

Maat Arija, Palmen Saskia. 2018. "Autismespectrumstoornis" In Handboek schizofreniespectrumstoornissen, edited by Wiepke Cahn, Inez Myin-Germeys, Richard Bruggeman, Lieuwe de Haan. Amsterdam: De Tijdstroom.

CHAPTER 31

ADHD

When is the ADHD classification met?

Almost everyone sometimes suffers from concentration problems or does something impulsive. But that does not mean that you suffer from attention deficit hyperactivity disorder, or ADHD. A characteristic of ADHD is that these symptoms persist for years and in an annoying way.

For the DSM-5 ADHD classification, there must be a persistent pattern of attention deficit (the DSM-5 refers to inattention) and / or hyperactivity-impulsivity. Some of the symptoms must have started before the age of twelve and are currently still bothersome. Due to the inattention and / or the hyperactivity, there must be dysfunction at school and at home.

The attention problems are:

1. Often fails to pay sufficient attention to details or makes careless mistakes in (school) work or other activities.
2. Often has trouble paying attention to tasks or play.
3. Often does not seem to listen when spoken to directly.
4. Often fails to follow directions and often fails to complete schoolwork, or work.
5. Often has difficulty organizing tasks and activities.
6. Often avoids or dislikes tasks that require sustained mental effort.
7. Often loses things necessary for tasks or activities (for example, toys, homework, pencils, books, or tools).
8. Often easily distracted by external stimuli.
9. Often forgetful about daily activities.

The symptoms of hyperactivity are:

1. Often fidgets with hands or feet, or turns in his / her chair.
2. Often stands up in class or in other situations where one is expected to remain seated.

3. Often runs around or climbs up in situations where it is inappropriate (in adolescents or adults, this may be limited to a feeling of restlessness).
4. Difficult to play or engage in quiet play
5. Is often "on the go" or "trundles on".
6. Talk often continuously.
7. Often throws out the answer before the question is fully asked.
8. Often has difficulty waiting his / her turn.
9. Often disrupts the activities of others or imposes himself on him (for example, just getting involved in conversations or games).

Children should only be classified as ADHD if they have at least six of the nine attention problems and / or six of the nine hyperactive / impulsive characteristics. Adults must meet four of the attention problems and / or five of the characteristics of hyperactivity or impulsivity.

Are there different forms of ADHD?

The most common form is the one with all three main symptoms: attention deficit, hyperactivity and impulsive behavior. Attention problems and impulsive behavior in particular often remain unchanged. Hyperactivity may diminish over time, but many patients whose hyperactivity is not immediately noticeable still experience inner turmoil or agitation.

Another form is ADHD with only attention problems (Attention Deficit Disorder, abbreviated to ADD). These are dreamy, introverted children or adults, easily distracted, but not busy or impulsive. ADD may be more common in girls. Smart children can often hide their problems with attention and concentration for a long time, until too high demands are placed on them in work or study.

Finally, ADHD is distinguished with only hyperactivity / impulsivity. This type is the least common.

How common is ADHD in children and adults?

About 3 to 5 percent of children ever meet the criteria for ADHD. ADHD is three to four times more common in boys than in girls. About 20 percent of children with ADHD still suffer from a single ADHD phenomenon in adulthood. About 30 percent of children with ADHD continue to suffer from ADHD into adulthood and continue to meet the criteria for ADHD. It follows that about 1 to 1.5 percent of adults meet the criteria for ADHD.

What is the treatment of ADHD?

It is important that patients learn to understand how the problems arose. This can decrease the degree of self-blame. In addition, it helps if partners and family understand better what the problem is. Medication is often prescribed for ADHD. Drugs of choice are methylphenidate (inhibits the reuptake of dopamine and norepinephrine, making these neurotransmitters active for a longer period in the synapse) and dextro-amphetamine (increases dopamine release). When someone with a vulnerability to develop psychosis needs farmacological treatment of ADHD than methylphenidate is preferred, since the risk on psychosis is higher with dextro-amphetamine. Both stimulate the dopamine system. It is believed that with ADHD the dopamine release is too low, so that people cannot concentrate properly. In about 70 percent of children and adults with ADHD, the first options have a beneficial effect on concentration, hyperactivity, impulsivity and aggressiveness. Stopping alcohol and drug use can reduce anxiety.

Are there other medications that can be prescribed for ADHD?

Another possible drug treatment of ADHD symptoms is the antidepressant desipramine, which inhibits the reuptake of noradrenaline (a neurotransmitter). Clonidine, a drug that is normally given to lower blood pressure, is also prescribed for ADHD. Desipramine and clonidine have less effect on improving concentration than the first drugs of choice, but a good effect has been found on hyperactivity, irritability and impulsivity.

Is treatment with medication wise for someone with a psychosis and ADHD?

Boosting dopamine can lead to overstimulation. This is probably not a good idea if someone has also suffered from a psychosis: especially treatment with dextro-amphetamine may be a triggering factor for a psychosis. However, little research has been done on this. There are case studies describing patients with ADHD and psychosis who are treated with a combination of antipsychotics and methylphenidate. A number of child and adolescent psychiatrists stated in a survey that this did not cause any problems. However, the safety and effectiveness of this combination of medications has not been sufficiently researched. Other contraindications (a contraindication is a compelling reason not to use a certain treatment) for methylphenidate or dextro-amphetamine are: epilepsy, cardiac arrhythmias, high blood pressure, an overactive thyroid gland, addiction and pregnancy. In short, prescribing drugs that stimulate dopamine to someone with a psychosis and ADHD is on the one hand accelerating, while on the other hand you have to brake.

Psychotherapeutic interventions in ADHD have not been sufficiently researched. Practice has shown that help with organizing and maintaining structure is often necessary.

CHAPTER 32

PERSONALITY TRAITS

What is meant by schizotype?

Schizotype is a particular personality trait that is on a continuum with schizophrenia. This is in line with the idea that vulnerability to psychiatric problems gradually distributed. It's not all or nothing, but more or less. A distinction is made between positive schizotypy (disturbances of thinking or perception, such as relational ideas, delusional experiences and brief hallucinatory experiences) and negative schizotypy (flattening of affect and social withdrawal). Family members of people with schizophrenia have higher levels of positive and negative schizotype. It was also found that there was a correspondence between the symptoms of patients with schizophrenia and the severity of schizotype in relatives. In recent research, schizotype is often considered to have psychosis-like symptoms or to display psychosis sensitivity or subclinical symptoms. A problem in measuring these phenomena is that it is often unclear whether they are stable personality traits or changeable phenomena.

What is the Five Factor Model of Personality Traits?

This concerns five basic personality traits:

1. neuroticism (the degree of sensitivity to negative emotions);
2. extraversion (the degree of outward directed energy);
3. openness (the degree of openness to new ideas and experiences);
4. altruism (the degree of orientation towards others);
5. conscientiousness (the degree of discipline, rigor and reliability).

Do the scores on the five-factor model differ between people with schizophrenia and people without a psychiatric illness?

In the five-factor model, people with schizophrenia score higher on average on neuroticism and lower on extraversion, openness, altruism and conscientiousness.

Are the abnormal scores on personality traits already present before schizophrenia is diagnosed?

Whether abnormal scores on personality traits are already present before schizophrenia is diagnosed is unknown. There are indications, however, that a higher score on neuroticism makes someone more vulnerable to develope psychosis. We do not know whether it is possible to reduce neuroticism, for example by learning to reduce stress. We also don't know whether reducing neuroticism reduces the risk of developing psychosis. We now think that personality traits can contribute to vulnerability as well as to resilience.

Are the scores on the five-factor model of people with schizophrenia just as stable as those of people without a psychiatric illness?

The neuroticism score in people with schizophrenia is associated with changes in negative and depressive symptoms and is less stable than in people without a psychiatric illness. This indicates that the degree of neuroticism also depends on a person's current state: when you are depressed or exhausted, you are naturally more sensitive to negative emotions.

Can the scores on the five-factor model of people with schizophrenia be used to select the most appropriate treatment?

One study found that a higher level of conscientiousness was predictive of the effectiveness of cognitive behavioral therapy. The degree of extraversion predicted the effectiveness of an interpersonal skills training. So far, only a few findings support the use of personality traits in treatment choice, but more research is desirable.

CHAPTER 33

METABOLIC SYNDROME

What is Metabolic Syndrome?

This is a condition in which there is a combination of several characteristics: excessive adipose tissue in the abdominal area, high blood pressure, reduced level of beneficial cholesterol and high blood fat levels, and a reduced ability to store sugar in the cell. The metabolic syndrome increases the risk of cardiovascular disease and diabetes.

What are the criteria for the metabolic syndrome?

If someone meets three or more of the criteria below, then you speak of a metabolic syndrome:

1. Excessive adipose tissue in the abdominal area, evidenced by a waist circumference of at least 94 cm in men and at least 80 cm in women
2. Decreased HDL cholesterol levels (HDL is a favorable form of cholesterol): less than 40 mg per deciliter of blood in men and less than 50 mg per deciliter of blood in women;
3. Elevated triglyceride levels of at least 150 mg per deciliter of fasting blood;
4. High blood pressure, with the upperlevel pressure [systolic] is at least 130 mm Hg and the lowerlevel pressure [diatolic] is at least 85 mm Hg;
5. Increased fasting blood sugar of at least 100 mg per deciliter of blood.

Why is the metabolic syndrome important?

The metabolic syndrome is important because it is one of the factors that contribute to premature death from cardiovascular disease. The main factor causing cardiovascular disease (and many other serious illnesses) is smoking. The great thing about factors such as metabolic syndrome or smoking is that you can basically influence them.

How often do modifiable risk factors for cardiovascular disease occur in people with schizophrenia?

Modifiable risk factors for cardiovascular disease occur in people with schizophrenia:

45 to 55 percent overweight;
Smoking at 50 to 80 percent;
Diabetes in 10 to 15 percent;
High blood pressure in 19 to 58 percent;
Increased blood fat levels in 25 to 69 percent.

During the first psychosis, about 10 percent of patients meet the definition of metabolic syndrome. Over time, this increases to about 35 percent of patients with schizophrenia.

Why is it that risk factors for cardiovascular disease are so common in people with schizophrenia?

The fact that risk factors for cardiovascular disease are so common in people with schizophrenia is partly due to unhealthy habits such as smoking, reduced physical activity and unhealthy eating (high in sugars and saturated fatty acids). In addition, treatment with antipsychotics can also have an unfavorable effect, especially with clozapine or olanzapine. It is less seen with aripiprazole. For a further discussion of these side effects, see Chapter 41 on Antipsychotics.

What causes obesity in people with schizophrenia?

Obesity can be caused by lack of exercise (which in turn can be caused by negative or depressive symptoms) and by increased appetite as a side effect of antipsychotics.

What weight gain increases the risk of physical disorders?

If an adult gains 7 percent weight, this is seen as a potential risk for physical disorders.

How is weight gain associated with antipsychotic use?

Between 15 percent and 72 percent of people with schizophrenia have a weight gain of 7 percent or more during antipsychotic treatment. Most weight gain occurs in people who are being treated with antipsychotics for the first time. Often the weight increases rapidly during the first weeks of treatment after which the increase gradually diminishes, usually reaching a plateau in the first year of treatment. The first weeks of treatment are therefore decisive. However, it is important to note that there are striking differences in weight gain between people treated with the same antipsychotic. Some have weight loss, while others gain tens of pounds. These differences are likely due to genetic variation.

How come antipsychotics can cause weight gain?

In the first place by increasing the appetite and in the second place by reducing the satiety signal. Therefore, you start more often with eating and go on with eating longer. The inhibitory effect of antipsychotics, especially clozapine and olanzapine, on certain serotonin and histamine receptors is probably responsible for this.

Can antipsychotics cause blood fat abnormalities?

Antipsychotic drugs may cause elevation of triglycerides and lowering of HDL cholesterol. These effects occur even before weight gain occurs.

Can Antipsychotics Cause High Blood Pressure?

The effect of antipsychotics on blood pressure is probably not very substantial. However, antipsychotics that inhibit certain adrenergic receptors may cause blood pressure to rise.

Can Antipsychotics Cause High Blood Sugar?

Antipsychotics increase the risk of developing diabetes. Olanzapine and clozapine in particular, and to a lesser extent quetiapine and risperidone, can cause elevated blood glucose levels. This may be due to the influence of clozapine and olanzapine in particular on the muscarinic receptors. This could disrupt the release of insulin and thus increase the sugar level in the blood.

What Is Diabetic Ketoacidosis?

This is a rare but serious acute disorder that can occur during diabetes. There is an absolute insulin deficiency, which causes the blood sugar level to be greatly increased, the blood becomes acidic and ketones enter the blood and urine. When this happens, you feel sick and sleepy, have a stomach ache and vomit. Usually, patients have fast breathing that smells sweet, are very thirsty and have to urinate often and a lot.

Diabetic ketoacidosis can seldom develop shortly after starting the use of clozapine and olanzapine.

What screening for cardiovascular risk factors is needed in patients with schizophrenia?

A profile of cardiovascular risk factors should be made in patients with schizophrenia. On the one hand, things like weight, blood fat and cholesterol, and blood sugar and blood pressure must be measured. On the other hand, risk factors such as unhealthy eating habits, smoking and little physical activity must be identified. This risk profile also includes information about personal and family history with regard to high blood pressure, cardiovascular disease and diabetes.

Children, adolescents and first-episode patients are especially at risk of developing metabolic syndrome and should be closely and frequently monitored during the first treatment period.

Why is waist measurement important?

The circumference of the abdomen depends on the amount of abdominal fat tissue and is related to the sensitivity of the body to insulin and therefore also to the blood sugar level. The circumference of the abdomen predicts the risk of diabetes better than the weight. In addition, the circumference of the abdomen is related to blood pressure and unhealthy blood fat levels. For these reasons, measuring abdominal circumference is the easiest way to determine the risk of metabolic syndrome.

How much effect has lifestyle change on health?

Quitting smoking, cutting back on salt, losing weight and more exercise can lower blood pressure and blood sugar levels. This reduces the risk of cardiovascular disease (heart attack or stroke). For example, if the diastolic blood-pressure drops from 90 mm Hg to 85 mm Hg, the risk of a heart attack decreases by 16 percent and the risk of a stroke by 42 percent. Better eating habits also have a significant effect on health. A 5 to 7 percent weight loss reduces the risk of diabetes by 58 percent. If a person maintains her ideal body weight, the risk of developing cardiovascular disease decreases by 35 to 60 percent. Quitting smoking reduces the risk of cardiovascular disease by 70 percent. More exercise improves health, even if no weight loss occurs. For example, walking briskly for half an hour every day reduces the risk of diabetes by 33 to 50 percent and the risk of cardiovascular disease by 27 percent.

For further benefits of exercise, see the section on physical activity.

CHAPTER 34

MOVEMENT DISORDERS

Are movement disorders always caused by antipsychotic drugs?

Movement disorders are not always caused by antipsychotics. There are also patients who have never used antipsychotics and who still suffer from movement disorders. Movement disorders can also be a symptom of schizophrenia. There are indications that movement disorders that occur without use of antipsychotics are an unfavorable sign. More severe cognitive problems and a less good response to antipsychotics were found in patients with movement disorders not caused by antipsychotics.

Which movement disorders can be caused by antipsychotics?

We can divide movement disorders into acute movement disorders, which develop within days of starting or increasing the dose of an antipsychotic (such as parkinsonism or akathisia), and into tardive movement disorders (tardus means late), which take months or years to develop (such as tardive dyskinesia and tardive dystonia).

Which medications can cause acute movement disorders?

All drugs that inhibit dopamine can cause acute movement disorders. These are usually antipsychotics, but also anti-vomiting agents and some antidepressants can cause movement disorders.

What is Acute Dystonia?

Dystonia is a spasm of one or more muscles that causes abnormal posture of the head, neck, limbs and / or trunk. Acute dystonia is often painful and distressing. Acute dystonia mainly occurs in muscles of the head and neck area. It can lead to a tilt of the head, a cramp in the muscles of the jaw, or around the eyes (the eyes turn in one direction, usually upwards) and cramping of the swallowing muscles. Acute dystonia can be extremely painful.

When can acute dystonia develop?

Nowadays, few patients suffer from acute dystonia. This is because fortunately lower doses of antipsychotics are being prescribed than before. But if it occurs, it almost always happens within the first four days of starting or increasing the dose of drugs that inhibit dopamine. The risk of acute dystonia is lower with an antipsychotic that does not inhibit dopamine very strongly. Recent cocaine use before starting an antipsychotic increases the risk of acute dystonia. Young patients have a markedly increased risk of acute dystonia.

How can you prevent acute dystonia?

You can prevent the development of acute dystonia by building up antipsychotics very gradually and by giving a less potent dopamine inhibitor. If someone is taking a potent dopamine inhibitor for the first time, it is wise to add an anticholinergic for about one week to prevent acute dystonia..

How Is Acute Dystonia Treated?

Acute dystonia is unpleasant or painful. That's why you want to get it treated quickly. This can be done with an anticholinergic, preferably intramuscularly (biperiden 5 mg), because the effect then occurs within 15 minutes. You can also take biperiden 5 mg by mouth, but it will take longer for the symptoms to ease. To prevent the dystonia from coming back, it is wise to keep taking anticholinergic drugs for at least two more days. If a person has spasms of the muscles around the eyes and anticholinergics do not help enough, then clonazepam can be tried.

What is Acute Akathisia?

Akathisia means "inability to sit." Visible symptoms are frequent crossing of the legs when someone has to sit and shift restlessly back and forth on a chair, wobbling with the legs or kicking with the feet, and always having to get up. In a queue, patients with akathisia often walk in place. Subjective complaints of akathisia are sometimes severe unpleasant feelings, usually in the legs but sometimes also in the abdomen. Those unpleasant feelings are described as restless, unpleasant and unbearable. Sometimes an unpleasant inner feeling precedes the akathisia. Akathisia is one of the most troublesome movement disorders, and of all movement disorders the main reason for non-adherence to therapy.

How often does akathisia occur and with which antipsychotics in particular?

Akathisia occurs in about 20-30 percent of patients on potent dopamine antagonists. Akathisia occurs frequently with aripiprazole or lurasidone, especially at the beginning of treatment. Akathisia can start as early as several hours after starting the antipsychotics.

How can you prevent akathisia?

Starting with a low dose and increasing it very gently can help prevent akathisia. In addition, the side effect is less common with antipsychotics that bind less strongly to the dopamine receptor (such as clozapine or quetiapine) and antipsychotics that already have an anticholinergic effect on their one (such as olanzapine).

How is akathisia treated?

The first step, to treat akathisia, is to lower the dose of the antipsychotic. If this does not help enough, a switch can be made to quetiapine, olanzapine or clozapine. Addition of a beta-blocker (for example propranolol 10 to 20 mg three times a day), mirtazapine 15 mg or an anticholinergic (the latter especially if symptoms of parkinsonism are present in addition to akathisia).

What does parkinsonism mean?

Parkinsonism consists of three symptoms that also occur in Parkinson's disease:

1. Little movement: patients suffer from general lack of movement and slowed movements, monotonous soft speech, little facial expression with a slightly open mouth, a bent posture, slow walking with small steps and a reduced arm swing.
2. Shaking, usually of the hands: This is also called the money counting tremor, because the shaking is like counting money. The head, legs and whole body can shake. With emotional stress, the shaking increases, and if someone performs a movement, the shaking can decrease.
3. Stiffness: patients suffer from stiffness of limbs and motor skills (due to increased muscle tension).

In addition to these visible symptoms, subjective symptoms also occur, such as loss of energy, fatigue, apathy, stiffness, slowness, clumsiness, coordination problems and easily tired and weakened muscles.

Parkinsonism can develop when more than 80 percent of dopamine receptors are occupied by an antipsychotic. The symptoms of Parkinson's disease only develop when more than 80 percent of the dopamine-producing cells have been lost. For that reason, the symptoms in Parkinson's disease do not improve over time: the lost cells do not return. Fortunately, parkinsonism due to antipsychotic drugs does improve when the dose of antipsychotics is reduced or when an antipsychotic is given that blocks dopamine receptors less strongly.

These symptoms usually occur at the beginning of the treatment with an antipsychotic. If the occupancy rate decreases, for example through dose reduction, the parkinsonism decreases or disappears. However, parkinsonism can also occur in patients who have never used antipsychotics. Parkinsonism is associated with an increased risk of tardive dyskinesia (see below).

How is Parkinsonism Treated?

If parkinsonism develops during treatment with an antipsychotic, then dose reduction of the antipsychotic is the obvious treatment. If an antipsychotic has been given that strongly adheres to the dopamine receptor (e.g., haloperidol or risperidone) and further dose reduction is not desirable, it may also help to switch to an antipsychotic that attaches less forcefully to the dopamine receptor (e.g. quetiapine or clozapine). Adding an anticholinergic appears to be much less effective than previously thought. In addition, anticholinergics have their own side effects, such as an increased risk of dry mouth, blurred vision, difficulty urinating and constipation.

What is myoclonus?

Myoclonus are sudden, jerky, involuntary movements. If myoclonus occurs once a day, this is normal, for example just before falling asleep. Hiccups are also a kind of myoclonic contraction. Myoclonus can be caused by antidepressants or clozapine, among others. Lowering the dose often helps.

What is Tardive Dyskinesia?

Tardive dyskinesia is an involuntary, twisting, repetitive movement of the muscles in the face (usually around the mouth), trunk, or limbs. Tardive means late. Tardive dyskinesia develops in the long run. Tardive dyskinesia is characterized by twisting movements of the tongue (where the tongue sometimes comes out of the mouth), smacking of the lips, chewing movements and frequent blinking of the eyes. Dyskinesia is striking, and many patients are ashamed of it.

What are risk factors for developing tardive dyskinesia?

The main risk factor for the development of tardive dyskinesia is the use of high doses of antipsychotics that bind vigorously to dopamine receptors. In those cases, tardive dyskinesia occurs in about 3 to 5 percent of patients. With antipsychotics that bind more loosely, this side effect occurs in 1 to 2 percent of patients. Other risk factors for developing tardive dyskinesia are older age, black ethnicity and parkinsonism during antipsychotic treatment.

These risk factors must be taken into account when choosing an antipsychotic.

How Is Tardive Dyskinesia Treated?

The first step in the treatment of tardive dyskinesia is to reduce the dose or (if justified) to discontinue the antipsychotic medication, or switching to a less potent antipsychotic (less strongly adhering to the dopamine receptor, e.g. clozapine).

If this does not help, treatment with tetrabenazine may be considered in severe tardive dyskinesia. However, it is important to be alert to depressive symptoms, which occur in 5 to 15 percent of the patients who use tetrabenazine. A high dose of vitamin E appeared to be successful in a number of small studies, but no effect was found in a large study in patients with long-term tardive dyskinesia. Perhaps a high dose of vitamin E can help if tardive dyskinesia recently started. There are also some indications that taking ginkgo biloba together with antipsychotics has a beneficial effect.

What is tardive dystonia?

An abnormal body posture caused by sustained muscle contractions is called tardive dystonia. This usually involves twisting of the neck or spasms of the muscles around the eyes. It can develop during treatment with antipsychotics or shortly after stopping their use. Tardive dystonia is less common than tardive dyskinesia and appears to occur mainly in chronic hospitalized patients. The risk factors for tardive dystonia are probably the same as those for tardive dyskinesia.

How is tardive dystonia treated?

The first step in the treatment of tardive dystonia is dose reduction or discontinuation of the antipsychotic, or a switch to clozapine. If this is not possible or desirable, a switch can be made to quetiapine.

What is Catatonia?

Catatonia is classified in the DSM-5 if someone experiences three or more catatonia symptoms. The main catatonic symptoms are:

1. Stupor: a condition in which someone is almost completely motionless with a clear consciousness and does not respond to stimuli from the environment.
2. Catalepsy: maintaining an unusual or unnatural posture for a long time, sometimes even for minutes.
3. Rigidity: Persistent rigid body posture despite attempts by others to induce movement. For example, you cannot or with difficulty bend someone's arm.
4. Flexibilitas cerea: limbs remain in the position in which the researcher placed them for a long time.
5. Mutism: virtually no speech or hardly any response.
6. Stare: fixed gaze.
7. Negativism: Refusing assignments without clear motive.
8. Hyperactivity / agitation: extreme activity or aggression, not caused by external stimuli.
9. Autonomous instability: abnormalities in body temperature, pulse, blood pressure, rate of breathing or sweat production.
10. Grimacing: artificial, strange, exaggerated movements of the face that seem to occur automatically
11. Echolalia: the unsolicited repetition of words.
12. Echopraxia: the unsolicited imitation of movements or facial expressions.
13. Stereotype: repetitive, aimless movements.
14. Perseveration: the continuous useless repetition of certain themes, phrases or actions.
15. Ambitendention: being motorically trapped in an indecisive, doubting movement, for example sitting down and getting up again immediately.

In which conditions does catatonia occur?

Catatonia can occur with mood disorders, physical disorders or schizophrenia.

Are there different forms of catatonia?

Four subtypes of catatonia are distinguished:

1. Stuporous catatonia: this concerns almost complete motionlessness, mutism and little or no response to external stimuli.
2. Catatonia with arousal state: patients exhibit excessive mobility, confusion, incoherent speech and disorientation. The picture can look very much like a delirious state or a mania.
3. Malignant catatonia: this serious condition develops acutely and is accompanied by fever and instability of the autonomic nervous system. Blood tests often show increased creatinine phosphokinase (an enzyme released when muscle or other cell damage occurs), increased white blood cells and decreased iron. The condition is very similar to neuroleptic malignant syndrome.
4. Periodic catatonia: These are recurring periods of catatonia that may be associated with abnormalities in the thyroid hormone and nitrogen balance.

How is Catatonia Treated?

Drug treatment of the stuporous form of catatonia begins with lorazepam

2-4 mg per day. If necessary, this is increased to 8-16 mg / day, provided that no unacceptable side effects develop. This is effective in about 80 percent of the cases. If after a few days it appears that drug treatment has no effect, then electroconvulsive therapy may be indicated. The motionlessness in severe catatonia increases the risk of blood clots. This can be a lifethreatening complication. Therefore, in case of persistent severe motionlessness, anticoagulant medication should be prescribed. In addition, in case of catatonia, consideration should be given to prescribing antipsychotics that bind less strongly to the dopamine receptors, because this type of antipsychotics can enhance catatonia symptoms.

PART 7.

TREATMENT

CHAPTER 35

PERSONAL RECOVERY

What is meant by personal recovery?

Personal recovery is about what people do to get back to life despite the consequences of their condition. When you are recovering, your self-image changes, you think about what you want to do and regain your faith in your own abilities. Recovery is related to feeling included in a social environment and being able to do what you want to do and find important. That way you can gradually regain faith and leave illness and stigma behind. Recovery can begin while you are still suffering from symptoms of the condition. Recovery does not mean that you no longer experience limitations. It means that you can and want to go on.

Most people who experience an accident, trauma, or illness try to get up again. Sometimes there are things that bother you, but when you recover you try to find new ways. However, recovery is by no means always easy. Either way, it makes sense to focus on your strengths, preferences, hobbies and talents. On the things that you really find valuable. However, some people with schizophrenia do not feel included in the social environment and are lonely and suspicious. Sometimes they are completely unable to do what they want and find important because they quickly become over-stimulated. This can make them desparate. Others can help you overcome these difficulties: you don't have to do it all alone. Personal recovery is in line with a new definition of health.

What does this new definition of health entail?

Health is the ability to adapt and take control of life's physical, emotional and social challenges. Being healthy means being able to adapt to disruptions, having resilience, maintaining or regaining a balance in physical, mental and social areas. This definition is therefore mainly about finding resilience and balance. In this definition, health is not the lack of disease symptoms. You can be bothered by something, but if you deal with it resiliently and if you find a new balance, then you are healthy. Yet this does sound very optimistic. People with schizophrenia often experience that they are not healthy. They have a vulnerability (or illness) and try to deal with it properly. It takes effort to reconcile with limitations. That is quite a job. It can be difficult that in addition to being resilient, you can also be (very) vulnerable and suffer a lot from a condition or disease.

Why is the attitude of the professional caregiver important to the recovery process?

If people with mental illness have suffered from “the rigid and limiting sides of psychiatric care,” they experience more stigma. As a result, people also tend to stigmatize themselves. If you stigmatize yourself and experience a lot of discrimination, you can lose faith. If care providers don’t take their patients ‘strengths seriously, it can diminish patients’ confidence in recovery. Sometimes counselors see patients’ ideas as a sign of the disorder and tend not to take them seriously. By intervening in these situations, because they believe that the patient is in danger, care providers can actually hinder recovery. Of course, it can also be a tricky business: not all people’s ideas lead to a new and favorable balance. Sometimes ideas actually involve significant risks. It is important that care providers try to make a good assessment together with patients. There is tension in this consultation: if the care provider estimates that the risks are too great, then she is inclined to take a paternalistic position. From the perspective of the recovery vision, this can only be justified if the risks are really overwhelming.

Which three dimensions of recovery are distinguished?

Four dimensions of recovery are distinguished:

1 recovery of health;
2 recovery of social functioning;
3 restoration of personal psychological identity.

What is meant by empowerment?

Empowerment means regaining autonomy and daring to take risks and responsibility.

You are captain of your own ship. Seeking advice and support from others can be a good fit for someone who has autonomy.

What are the underlying ideas of the recovery movement?

People with severe psychiatric illness often have unsuspected strengths and talents that are worthwhile. Taking control, emancipation, empowerment and self-determination is essential. Everyone has limitations. Everyone must take this into account. Everyone depends on others. Future dreams are translated into achievable goals in the short term. Taking risks is sometimes unavoidable here. If you go faster than you can handle, you can lose your balance. Learning the difference between responsible and irresponsible risks is an important goal of recovery. Timing is important here: if you are doing well, you can sometimes take risky steps, but during crises it is better to play it safe. Experiential expertise is of great importance here.

What four questions can help with the recovery process?

1. What happened to you?
2. What is your vulnerability and what is your resilience?
3. Where do you want to go?
4. What do you need? (And who do you need?)

The great thing about these questions is that anyone can ask them themselves. Moreover, these questions are not only about illness and vulnerability, but about normal life, about your life. Sometimes people without so-called serious problems take a long time to find good answers. The questions are simple, but they are about valuable things. They help you to find your own position and to build up awareness of your resilience and your limitations, and to clarify what you want, what you want to develop yourself and what help you need from other people.

CHAPTER 36

FUNCTIONAL RECOVERY, REHABILITATION AND STIGMA

What is Functional Recovery and Rehabilitation?

Functional recovery is about resuming living, learning, working, contacts, relationships and activities. Rehabilitation helps people with severe difficulties to function better so that they can live, work, learn and socialize successfully and happily, with as little professional help as possible. On the one hand, this is done by offering them care to promote participation in society. On the other hand, rehabilitation represents a social movement that strives for the emancipation of patients. Rehabilitation is closely related to beliefs about recovery. A side note: in recent decades, people with psychological vulnerability have been expected to be as self-reliant as possible and to rely on their "own strength". It is important for politicians to realize that, in addition to their own strength, there is also vulnerability, and that people with schizophrenia must be able to rely on good care and support.

Why rehabilitation?

Many people with schizophrenia have a small social network. About 75 percent of them often feel lonely. 80 percent live alone. Only about 10 to 20 percent of people with schizophrenia are in paid employment and only about 25 to 50 percent have unpaid work or daytime activities. And that's not what most people with schizophrenia want: the majority would like to have more contact with others, about 70 percent would like to be more active, and about 70 percent of people who are out of work would like to work. Rehabilitation can help them change this.

What are the causes of social isolation of many people with schizophrenia?

Social isolation can be caused by severe symptoms, limited skills, and lack of experience. But it can also be due to unfavorable circumstances, such as a low income, little social support, long hospital stays and difficulty in finding a suitable place to live. There are also annoying social circumstances, such as stigmatization and complicated regulations. In addition, there is also relatively little work available adapted to vulnerable groups.

When to start rehabilitation?

Rehabilitation should begin right at the start of treatment. When you are about twenty and you develop psychosis, you care about continuing your further education, looking for work, start living independently and fall in love. Your goals should be at the top of the agenda from the start of early intervention in psychosis. Social and professional recovery immediately after a first psychosis predicts a more favorable outcome. Of course, all of these things should not be addressed at the same time. Phasing is needed.

Doing too much will quickly make you sicker in the middle of a psychosis. But recovery and rehabilitation is of utmost importance for people who have been suffering from a psychotic disorder. Finally, it should also remain a priority in older patients. That is why it is important that there are opportunities for social activities.

Why is rehabilitation of the people most affected by severe psychiatric illness so important?

Often people who live in a psychiatric institution or sheltered housing for a long time were seen as patients for whom there was no improvement. It was only about accepting that situation. As a result, the professional caregiver contributed to loss of identity and isolation. Everyone needs hope. You need a future. We need to look at what is still possible.

Rehabilitation is therefore important in treatment for both people with schizophrenia in sheltered housing and for patients living independently. There are several approaches to rehabilitation, some of which are discussed below.

What does the individual rehabilitation approach look like?

In the individual rehabilitation approach, a clear distinction is made between treatment (with an emphasis on minimizing disease symptoms) and rehabilitation (with an emphasis on maximizing health). There are modules for learning and social contacts.

This approach has a phase model: exploring, choosing, and then obtaining or retaining. First, together with the patient, it is determined what her goal is and what skills and what support are needed to achieve that goal. Then the necessary interventions and skills training are selected and carried out. Randomized controlled research shows that patients with this method themselves notice that they achieve their goals more often and that it leads to more social participation. Rehabilitation is based on the strength of people.

What are the Liberman modules?

The Liberman modules are about learning skills and coping strategies. Treatment and rehabilitation overlap. They are group skills training, based on the principles of social learning and with a lot of emphasis on a step-by-step approach and behavioral practice. Training courses include living skills, care, leisure, work, social relationships and intimacy. The advantage is that you also learn from each other in a group and that it is more fun than working on your own. These training courses have not been investigated for effectiveness.

What is the disadvantage of such group training?

The disadvantage of these group training courses is that transferring the skills learned in the training to everyday life is difficult. To achieve that, the training must teach you skills that you can use immediately. Practicing for later doesn't work. In addition, exercise is most effective in a situation that is very similar to everyday life. In addition, to learn to apply new skills, you need the support of someone important to you.

What is Cognitive Remediation?

Cognitive remediation focuses on improving cognitive functioning through exercises (usually on the computer). This intervention appears to be effective, but must go hand in hand with other forms of rehabilitation.

What is Cognitive Adaptation Training?

Cognitive Adaptation Training (CAT) does not focus on improving cognitive functioning, but on compensating for cognitive impairments by developing compensation strategies. The effectiveness of this training has been demonstrated.

What is Individual Placement and Support?

Because step-by-step processes (first training and then placement) are less effective and can have a demotivating effect, Individual Placement and Support (IPS) has been developed. IPS assumes that any patient who wishes to do so, can work in a regular workplace with supervision. Participants are quickly placed in the chosen position and then trained in the necessary work skills (first place, then train). The IPS counselor is also part of the treatment team. Research in several countries showed that IPS is very successful: about 60 percent of the participants in IPS got a regular job, compared to 20 percent of the people who received other work interventions. Many people will also keep their jobs in the longer term. A good number of them even have an upward trend in their career.

What is stigma?

People with schizophrenia experience discrimination in social contacts, in the family, in intimate relationships and at work. Many people prefer not to have a psychiatric patient as a neighbor, employee, colleague, friend, partner or son/daughter-in-law. The idea that psychiatric patients are dangerous and unpredictable is persistent. In such a climate, it is understandable that many people hide that they have (or have had) psychiatric problems.

What is Self Stigma?

If people themselves had negative images of psychiatric patients before they had psychiatric problems, they then apply this to themselves. We call this self-stigma. As a result, they often don't even look for work or friendships, because they think they will be rejected anyway.

What can you do about stigma?

Protesting against stigma does not lead to a change in attitude of people in society, but it can counteract stigmatizing (media) statements. In educational materials, emotionally charged myths about mental illness can be debunked by facts. But this also does not cause a clearly more positive attitude in the population. What does seem to have an effect is encounters between patients and other citizens. During contact, citizens become acquainted with (former) patients. These interventions should be repeated and be a pleasant experience for all involved. It is most effective to apply this intervention with employers, police officers, teachers and local residents, because these people have a lot of impact on the lives of patients and have a lot of influence on others, respectively.

CHAPTER 37

FAMILY TREATMENT

What spectacular development in schizophrenia and psychosis care has taken place in the past 40 years?

The role of the family has changed radically. In the 1970s and 1980s, some professionals had a shameful and cruel explanation for schizophrenia: it was said to be caused by "the schizophrenogenic mother"! Now that crappy idea has disappeared. The mother and other loved ones are "allies" or "caregivers". In any case, family members play an active role in care.

No one is to blame anymore. That's a good thing, because blaming a guilty party is a malicious and primitive response. It does not make any sense. Of course, that does not mean that nothing ever goes wrong in families. The fact that you can do things wrong also applies to professional caregiver and to yourself. It happens that people within families suffer trauma. And it also happens that contact with family is not good for your recovery. But in the vast majority of cases, the family is very caring and involved. Fortunately, the realization has grown that you need family and that the professional caregiver and the family need each other.

Does family involvement have any beneficial effects?

Family involvement clearly has beneficial effects, research shows. Patients recover better if family members are actively involved in care. Patients from families who had a family intervention lived on average ten months less in a psychiatric residential facility than patients whose parents did not receive this family intervention. Patients with first psychosis whose relatives participated in family groups were about 50 percent less likely to have a psychotic relapse. These beneficial effects may have contributed to the fact that caring and involved family members dropped less often out of therapy. It is possible that things will get better anyway with patients who have caring and committed family members.

Family members often have more influence on the patient than their professional caregivers and can therefore help prevent coercion. If family members are involved in the treatment, patient satisfaction is higher. The relationship between patients and their relatives is then also better.

Why is family involvement so important?

People with psychosis or schizophrenia sometimes lose friends, acquaintances, colleagues or fellow students. They sometimes get fellow sufferers and therapists (who often change) in return. That is one of the reasons why the family remains so important. But not only for that: your family will always be your family. Your family provides social support, you are rooted there, that is often your home base. However, family is not always a safe home base. Then it is important to find others who are involved. We all need people who care and remain available.

Why is it so difficult for parents to balance commitment and letting go with their child with psychosis?

Parents are involved in parenting until about the eighteenth or twentieth year of life. After that, children are more and more independent. Parents let them go. But when children develop psychosis, parents tend to bring children back. Letting go is difficult then. Parents are concerned and scared. Sometimes rightly so, but sometimes parents simply cannot get rid of their concerns. Letting go normally means more or less the opposite of involvement. Here, however, by letting go I mainly mean: giving space to grow up. Psychotic children / young people sometimes need longer in this process and often also need more support. Sometimes it is never possible to stand on your own feet. Tension can arise about the degree of involvement: how much autonomy should parents give and how much support? How many things must parents learn to accept and how many demands are they allowed to make? And which rules apply at home? So extended upbringing and autonomy, but in what proportion? Young people with a psychosis have to resume their own development and ideally do not return home (for too long). Although that can sometimes be a good solution, though.

Why can "just being a family member" so difficult?

"Just being a family member" means continuing to do all normal family things. Celebrating Christmas, dividing the attention between your children. Live your own life, keep seeing your friends, go on holydays. But this may be difficult. About 65 percent of family members have difficulties with it. Worrying about your child with psychosis consumes you and costs energy. Other members of the family often struggle with it as well. Your child has changed and with that, family life has also changed, whether you like it or not. That is difficult and it takes time to adjust.

Why can informal care be such a difficult task?

Informal care is particularly difficult, because the responsibility remains, every day, sometimes for decades. It is therefore important to keep a good demarcation of tasks and a clear role for the professional care provider. One in eight informal carers is the only helper. One in five carers experiences a barrier to asking for support for themselves. Among the overburdened helpers, the helpers of people with a psychological problem are overrepresented.

What difficulties may patients have with their families?

Patients also sometimes run into problems with their families. For example, that your family wants more from you than you want. Or that your parents don't understand you. Or that you are convinced that your family is causing your problems. Or that your family gets angry or sad when you talk to them. Or that you are afraid of losing your parents. Or that you don't dare to ask for help from your family because they already did so much for you. Or that you feel alone because your brother or sister has children and a job and you don't.

If you are struggling with this, it generally helps to talk to someone about it, such as a friend, another family member, or your professional caregiver. Sometimes it can also help to bring it up in family conversations. When family members learn to understand each other's perspective and difficulties, a lot has already been gained.

CHAPTER 38

CONTACT WITH FELLOW SUFFERERS

Why can contact with fellow sufferers help you?

Humans are social beings. Many studies show that people do much better when they feel included in a group and when they feel understood. If you suffer from a psychosis, you will often be more alone. Sometimes people deliberately isolate themselves, sometimes they no longer dare to be among people, and sometimes it is too stressful to have contact with others. Contact with fellow sufferers can help. You are not alone. You notice how nice it is when someone else supports you and you notice how nice it is when you can do something for someone else. It is often pleasant to interact with more people. Of course, there can also be negative sides to contact with fellow sufferers. For example, you can't get along with everyone and you can worry about someone else. People can also have a less favorable influence on each other. But usually, the beneficial effects of contact with fellow sufferers predominate.

In general, is there a relationship between the social network and outcome in terms of symptoms and functioning?

A smaller social network is associated, according to a meta-analysis, with more severe general symptoms (effect size = 0.53) and more severe negative symptoms (effect size = -0.75). A correlation between the size of the social network and the severity of positive symptoms and social functioning was not found. It is important to realize that this is "only" an association. It is not certain that improving the social network will reduce symptoms. The link may be found because people with less severe general or negative symptoms have more energy to build a larger network.

What is the effect of one-on-one contact with fellow sufferers?

The effect of one-on-one contact with fellow sufferers was investigated in a randomized study in which 114 patients received a fellow sufferer plus normal treatment, and 102 patients only normal treatment. The expectations people have of their own skills (the belief in their own abilities) increased in the group with fellow sufferers. Quality of life, social functioning and hospital admissions did not differ between the two conditions.

Does peer contact help improve patients' healthy behavior and physical activity?

A systematic review article has been written about the effect of peer contact on healthy behavior and physical activity in patients. Seven small studies have been done. In six of these, no clear positive effects of peer contact on weight loss or on healthy behavior were found. One study found an increase in patient self-reported physical activity and healthier eating. In short, there is hardly any evidence that peer contact helps to promote healthy behavior.

Can peer contact via social media help?

Contact via social media has many advantages: you do not have to travel, you can use it at a time of your choice, it is fast, you can respond immediately and you can maintain friendship from a distance. You can find and support each other through specific groups.

Do interventions via social media have an effect?

A systematic review article shows that depressive symptoms decrease after using social media, but it has no effect on anxiety symptoms or psychotic symptoms. People accept these kinds of interventions, they continue to use social media and they are perceived as safe. However, studies with a control group are missing.

How do people with psychotic illness use social media?

A systematic review article shows that people with a psychotic illness use chat rooms more often and for longer and play games via the web more often than people without a psychosis. People with psychosis made less use of Facebook and e-mail.

How are ICT applications developed by fellow sufferers aimed at psychosis information and treatment used and experienced?

A review article shows that about 80 percent of patients make good use of web-based interventions aimed at psychosis information and treatment, about 85 percent find them useful and benefit from it. There are indications that these interventions can have beneficial effects on positive symptoms, social embedding, depression and medication adherence.

What is the effect of contact with fellow sufferers via the internet, without the involvement of a site manager?

A randomized controlled trial has been done on this. No difference in recovery, quality of life, social support or feelings of stress was found between the intervention condition (participation in online peer support group) and the control condition (no intervention). It was even found that more frequent participation in peer-to-peer contact increased the feeling of stress (although there were also more positive experiences). Perhaps unstructured peer contact via the internet can also be stressful.

CHAPTER 39

EARLY INTERVENTION IN PSYCHOSIS

Why was Early Intervention in Psychosis developed?

Early intervention was developed from the idea that early treatment in psychosis and early attention to improving functioning can improve the prognosis in the longer term.

Why focus on early intervention?

Many psychiatric disorders develop at an early age and early intervention yields improvement, and prevents development of more serious problems. Moreover, more and more attention is paid to outpatient care and to the extent to which longer duration of untreated psychosis negatively influences the outcome of treatment.

What is meant by the duration of untreated psychosis?

The duration of untreated psychosis (DUP) is the time that elapses between the onset of psychotic symptoms and initiation of adequate antipsychotic treatment. Sometimes the definition of DOP also assumes the onset of other important aspects of treatment, such as psychotherapy or rehabilitation. However, in most studies, the time when adequate antipsychotic medication treatment begins is seen as the endpoint of the untreated psychosis.

Is there a relationship between the duration of untreated psychosis and the short-term outcome?

A number of meta-analyzes have shown that the longer the DUP, the more severe the symptoms are at the time of the first treatment and that the severity of the symptoms subsequently decreases less well. Social functioning and quality of life are also worse at the start of treatment with a longer DUP.

Is there a relationship between the duration of untreated psychosis and the long-term outcome?

Meta-analyzes also showed that there is a relationship between DUP and long-term outcome. For example, it was found that the long-term severity of negative symptoms is larger in people who had a DUP of more than one year. No link was found between the DUP and having a job.

Could the relationship between the duration of untreated psychosis and outcome be explained by other factors?

There can, of course, be factors that influence the relationship between DUP and prognosis. For example, people who are less well off could start treatment later. It could then be that this third factor (having a worse prognosis anyway) is related to both DUP and the outcome. You call this confounding. It means that a third factor is related to both the predictive factor (DUP) and the outcome. This third factor disrupts the causal relationship between DUP and the outcome or is itself the basis for the relationship. Then the relationship between DUP and prognosis could possibly be caused by unfavorable factors that are present anyway and that are associated with DUP. This could prevent shortening the DOP from helping. After all, you do not improve the underlying factors that determine the prognosis. A meta-analysis investigated whether an important confounder (the level of functioning prior to the onset of psychosis) could explain the relationship between DUP and prognosis. That turned out not to be the case. However, other studies have found a link between the speed at which psychotic symptoms develop and DUP. It turned out that patients whose psychosis developed gradually started treatment later. That also sounds logical: an insidious start is less noticeable, and then the alarm is sounded later. But an insidious start is in itself associated with a less good prognosis.

What about the relationship between DUP and prognosis?

It is probably wisest to assume that some of the link between DUP and prognosis is due to factors associated with prognosis that do not improve with faster treatment. On the other hand, part of the relationship between DUP and prognosis seems to be determined by the causal effects of treatment delay. But you will only know for sure if you have investigated this in a randomized study with a control condition in which one group receives an early intervention and the other group a later intervention. But then you first have to check whether shortening the DUP is possible at all.

Is it possible to shorten the duration of untreated psychosis?

A recent meta-analysis showed that there is no effect of various interventions aimed at shortening the duration of untreated psychosis. It therefore turns out to be very difficult to treat groups of patients earlier. What we can do in any case is to treat patients with a first psychosis as quickly as possible. But specific interventions have not proven to be useful.

Does this invalidate the value of attempts to start treatment quickly?

This does not mean that the value of attempts to start treatment quickly, because it is worthwhile in any case to make the duration of psychotic symptoms as short as possible. The shorter you have been suffering from psychosis, the less impact it has on education, work and social functioning. Faster initiation of psychosis treatment also reduces the risk of aggression or suicide attempts.

What are important goals of Early Intervention in Psychosis?

Start treatment soon; Reduce treatment failure; Prevent suicide; Prevent admission; Promote symptomatic, functional and personal recovery; Provide information to patient and family to increase knowledge and a sense of control; Stop drug use or reduce use; Prevent new psychotic episode.

What are important features of Early Intervention in Psychosis?

Treatment of a first psychosis for a limited time (usually three to five years); Care is accessible and aimed at continuity; Multidisciplinary team and treatment offer; Outreach and outpatient care; Involving family in treatment; Focus on taking up training or work; Focus on what is possible.

Is there an optimal duration of Early Intervention in Psychosis?

There are indications that the course during the first three to five years of a psychotic illness is important for the long-term prognosis. There are no clear indications that intensive Early Intervention in Psychosis must necessarily last five years if the standard care that follows VIP is sufficiently good. Namely, there was no improvement in the primary outcome measure "negative symptoms" in a randomized controlled trial comparing the group that received five years of Early Intervention in Psychosis with a group that received two years of Early Intervention in Psychosis and three years of standard care. However, the members of the group with long-term Early Intervention in Psychosis more often had a lasting good cooperation with professional caregiver (90 percent versus about 56 percent) and were more satisfied.

If you succeed in completing education and / or finding stable meaningful structural activities (including, for example, work) in the first three to five years, then the likelihood of long-term symptomatic, functional and personal recovery is higher. Those first three to five years are labeled as a critical period. This means that the further course is influenced by how things are going in those first years. The fact that this is also referred to as a five-year critical period is because research into shorter-term interventions showed that improvements were partially lost after a longer period of time. Apparently intensive support was needed longer. Incidentally, it also turned out that for some patients even longer intensive care is required. Therefore, you could also say that three to five years of intensive care is enough for most people to discover how much recovery they can achieve and how much support they need. In individual cases, it is probably wisest to continue the care that appears to be needed in the final year of the "critical phase" in subsequent years. In this way, the critical period can be seen as a time in which it gradually becomes clear how much care is needed for the best possible symptomatic, functional and personal recovery.

What is the short-term effect of Early Intervention in Psychosis?

A meta-analysis was published of ten randomized studies in which a total of 2176 patients participated and in which the intervention lasted an average of 16.2 months. At the end of the treatment period, the outcome was better in the group receiving Early Intervention in Psychosis:

Fewer people dropped out (relative risk = 0.70, which means that if 100 patients stop standard care, 70 patients stop Early Intervention in Psychosis);

Fewer people had one or more psychiatric admissions (relative risk = 0.74, which means that if 100 patients in the standard care group are admitted one or more times, this will happen to 74 patients with Early Intervention in Psychosis);

More people went to school or work (relative risk = 1.13, meaning that if there are 100 patients in the standard care group going to school or work, there are 113 patients with Early Intervention in Psychosis who do this).

At the end of treatment, the severity of all symptoms together was less in the Early Intervention in Psychosis group than in the standard care group (effect size = -0.32). Positive symptoms (effect size = -0.22) and negative symptoms (effect size = -0.28) were also less severe in the Early Intervention in Psychosis treatment group.

What is the long-term effect of Early Intervention in Psychosis?

The beneficial effect at the end of Early Intervention in Psychosis treatment was maintained after 6, 9, 12, and 18 to 24 months of treatment. Only the effect on the severity of total and depressive symptoms between 18 and 24 months was not different between Early Intervention in Psychosis and standard treatment. Several studies have found that Early Intervention in Psychosis treatment effects remain demonstrable up to one and three years after the end of Early Intervention in Psychosis. Over time, however, there is a tendency to loose treatment effects. In short, there is some evidence that Early Intervention in Psychosis can help improve functioning, but a significant proportion of patients may require continued care to maintain these beneficial effects.

CHAPTER 40

PSYCHOEDUCATION

What does psychoeducation entail?

Psychoeducation is information about the development of psychiatric disorders and about the symptoms and their treatment. Initially, psychoeducation was provided only to the family and the emphasis was on the high risk of psychotic relapse and limited expectations regarding future functioning. Nowadays the content of psychoeducation is more optimistic and focused on recovery, getting to know one's own strengths and dealing with limitations. Psychoeducation for patients has broadly the same content as that for family members. This book is an example of psychoeducation (Van der molen A et al., 2018).

What is the purpose of psychoeducation?

The goal is for all involved to be able to cope better with the condition, or more specifically: Increase knowledge on psychoses; Increase knowledge of treatment options; Increase the problem-solving capacity of the patient and those close to them.

What questions should be addressed in psychoeducation?

What are psychotic symptoms? What does the diagnosis of schizophrenia entail? What are the treatment options? What is the expected course? Which factors influence the course? How can you reduce the risk of relapse? How can you learn to deal better with problems or limitations? What solutions are possible?

Does psychoeducation have a beneficial effect?

Psychoeducation aimed at the family and the patient reduces the risk of returing of the psychotic symptoms, improves the expertise of the family and improves mutual understanding and communication.

Why is psychoeducation important for patients?

If you suffer from symptoms that fall under the classification schizophrenia (or another schizophrenia spectrum disorder), this often has an impact on your expectations for the future. For example, can you complete your education, do you manage to find work and do you still find a partner? How much stress can you handle, how well can you concentrate?

On the one hand, discussing the classification schizophrenia does justice to the problems and the necessary professional help. On the other hand, discussing it can increase self-stigma, leaving you too little confidence in your resilience, and making you more depressed.

Good psychoeducation contributes to the necessary knowledge about your condition, which gives you a better grip on the factors that influence your vulnerability, but certainly also on factors that can increase your resilience. This way you can have the courage to focus on what you find important in your life and use your strengths (Van der molen A et al., 2018).

Why is psychoeducation important for close relatives?

Psychosis usually develops in adolescence, precisely when someone is on the way to independence. The classification of schizophrenia is not only difficult for patients to accept, but close relatives can also be sad, disappointed, worried or angry, or feel guilty. Parents and other loved ones often worry about the future. In addition, family members often also need advice on how to deal with certain difficulties. Family members can also experience support from each other when psychoeducation is given in groups.

References

Van der molen A et al., 2018. "Psychoeducate" In Handboek schizofreniespectrumstoornissen, edited by Wiepke Cahn, Inez Myin-Germeys, Richard Bruggeman, Lieuwe de Haan. Amsterdam: De Tijdstroom.

CHAPTER 41

ANTIPSYCHOTIC MEDICATION

Antipsychotics are an important part of the treatment options for psychotic symptoms. Whether and, if so, which antipsychotics are used (and in what dosage) should be decided together between you and your psychiatrist. Whether or not to start with an antipsychotic depends on the nature, severity and duration of the psychiatric problems.

The purpose of this chapter on antipsychotics is to familiarize patients and family members with the medical and scientific knowledge about antipsychotics. This knowledge allows you to agree on an optimal treatment strategy together with your professional caregiver. If you are more involved in that choice, then you also feel more responsible for it.

Finding the agent and optimal dosage is sometimes hard work. Much is known about the chance of an effect and the risk of side effects, but only by trying it out will it become clear how the drug works for you. That is why it can sometimes take quite some time to find the optimal antipsychotic medication.

Background

What is the history of antipsychotics?

A French surgeon noticed in 1956 that patients he had anaesthetized with chlorpromazine became indifferent. Then it was decided to give chlorpromazine to manic patients. They too calmed down. Subsequently, it turned out that people with schizophrenia were less confused when they took chlorpromazine. Many patients treated with chlorpromazine were able to return to society after years of residence in psychiatric institutions. The drug was also used in patients with tics and compulsive disorders. A short time later, the antipsychotics haloperidol and perphenazine were developed. Often patients treated with these agents suffered from severe parkinsonism (tremors, stiffness, walking with small steps) or acute dystonia (painful spasm in a muscle), because the dosage was too high.

In the late 1950s, clozapine was developed as an antidepressant. Later it turned out to be a very effective antipsychotic. It was striking that practically no parkinsonism or acute dystonia occurred with clozapine use. More than ten years after clozapine was marketed, its use became severely restricted, after a number of people died of infections due to a rare but serious side effect of clozapine. Their white blood cell count had fallen sharply. Since then, clozapine should only be prescribed with regular monitoring of the white blood cells.

After this, a search was made for antipsychotics that were as effective as clozapine, but did not have this rare serious side effect. Drugs such as olanzapine and quetiapine and risperidone entered the market and were called "atypical antipsychotics," "second-generation antipsychotics," or simply "new antipsychotics." Olanzapine and quetiapine are very similar to clozapine in chemical structure and the type of receptors on which they act. Still, they turned out not to be as effective as clozapine.

At the end of the last century, aripiprazole was developed: an antipsychotic with a new mode of action. It has both an inhibitory and a stimulating effect on the dopamine receptor.

What Are Antipsychotics?

Antipsychotics are drugs that have been shown to reduce psychotic symptoms. If research shows that a drug is effective in reducing psychotic symptoms and has acceptable side effects, it can be registered as an antipsychotic. All registered antipsychotics have a blocking effect on the dopamine receptor. This means that the antipsychotic binds on the dopamine receptor and blocks the action of dopamine on that receptor. This reduces the effect of dopamine. For a description of the influence of dopamine on the processing of information I refer to Chapter 19.

For what reasons are antipsychotics prescribed?

Antipsychotics are prescribed to reduce psychotic symptoms (delusions, hallucinations, and confusion). Antipsychotics can also be used when someone is manic or when there is danger or harm from being very impulsive or uninhibited.

In addition, antipsychotics are also prescribed to prevent recurrence of psychotic symptoms. This is called maintenance treatment. For example, if someone qualifies as having schizophrenia and has recovered from a second psychotic period on antipsychotics, it is wise to continue taking antipsychotics.

Not because someone still suffers from psychotic symptoms, but because the risk of a new psychosis in this case is high (at least 80 percent) and because antipsychotics help to reduce this risk. Long-term use of antipsychotics is often difficult to accept. To make it more acceptable, it is important that you use an antipsychotic in a dosage that causes as few side effects as possible.

What is the effect of antipsychotics?

Antipsychotics reduce the effect of dopamine and thus inhibit the importance you attach to an experience or a thought and the impact of that experience or thought on your behavior. So, you become somewhat more indifferent to experiences or thoughts. They hurt you less. This is the fundamental trait that all antipsychotics share. For example, if antipsychotics are given to patients who have unrealistic ideas that they attach too much importance to (called delusions), antipsychotics reduce the effect of dopamine, thereby reducing the importance people attach to these ideas. Your thoughts calm down. Likewise, antipsychotics reduce the importance attached to experiences, memories, or internal speech that are perceived as too impressive (hallucinations). The weight assigned to ideas and perceptions decreases, making people feel calmer.

How do antipsychotics work in the brain?

All antipsychotics inhibit the action of dopamine in the brain. They do this by binding to the dopamine receptor, so that dopamine can no longer stimulate this receptor. As a result, dopamine cannot send a signal to the next cell and the importance network in your brain calms down, thereby reducing delusions, hallucinations, excitement, aggression and fear. What dopamine does and what happens when the dopamine receptor is blocked is described in detail in Chapter 19.

Does it matter what percent of dopamine receptors are occupied by an antipsychotic?

If more than 80 percent of the dopamine receptors are occupied by an antipsychotic, then parkinsonism occurs: symptoms that also occur in Parkinson's disease, such as stiffness, tremors or reduced movement. These side effects disappear when the dose is lowered and the occupancy of dopamine receptors lowers below 80%. At an occupancy higher than 70 percent, subjective complaints can arise in some people. Some patients then feel muffled and inhibited. On the other hand, an occupancy that is clearly lower than 60 percent is associated with a less good effect on psychotic symptoms. So, there is an optimal occupancy: high enough to be effective, low enough not to cause subjective complaints and parkinsonism. This optimal occupancy is usually between 60 and 70 percent.

You can measure the occupancy of dopamine receptors by antipsychotics with SPECT and PET research, expensive specialist research that uses radioactive material. However, it is unwise to employ such techniques in normal clinical practice. In the first place, this research indicates radiation exposure, possibly acceptable in research, but undesirable in regular care, and secondly, it is too expensive and not feasible everywhere. For that reason, you determine the optimal dosage in consultation with your psychiatrist. Your experiences with the antipsychotic are guiding in this. The dose must be high enough to be effective and low enough to prevent or minimize parkinsonism and subjective side effects. That is customization. Usually, it is wise to start with a very low dose and then gradually increase it until an effect begins.

[By the way, there is a new way to visualize the amount of dopamine in your brain without using radiation. This can be done with a MRI scan for neuromelanine [a break-down product of dopamine]. Research shows that a neuromelanine MRI scan may be helpful in distinguishing patients who will have a good therapeutic response from those who are resistant to treatment with non-clozapine antipsychotics. Further research is needed.] (Knegtering R and Bruggeman R. 2018).

Does the speed with which the antipsychotic releases from the dopamine receptor have influence?

Quetiapine and clozapine are special antipsychotics and do not produce a high percentage of blockade, because they bind to the receptor for a relatively short time and release from it easily. This allows the naturally occurring dopamine to return to the receptor and have an effect. It is thought that this allows a more natural function of dopamine. Moreover, this explains why the side effect of parkinsonism is hardly seen with quetiapine and clozapine. The occupancy of dopamine receptors by quetiapine and clozapine never exceeds 80 percent. You might wonder why not everyone is treated with these drugs. That is because there are also some disadvantages to treatment with these drugs. See below.

What is meant by partial dopamine agonist?

Aripiprazole is a partial dopamine agonist. “Agonist” refers to stimulation. Aripiprazole thus partially stimulates the dopamine receptor. Partial dopamine agonists occupy a very high percentage of the dopamine receptors, but they not only inhibit but also act on the receptor similar to the effect that dopamine has. However, the effect is weaker than that of dopamine itself. The result is that the dopamine system is inhibited, but not completely, some activity remains. Herewith it is thought to obtain an optimal mix between inhibition and stimulation with aripiprazole.

Which antipsychotics are used and roughly in which dosage in adults?

The following antipsychotics (listed in alphabetical order) are generally used at the following doses (NB: sometimes lower or higher doses are indicated than described below):

Amisulpride. Start with 100 mg. Usually a dose between 200 and 800 mg is sufficient for a first psychosis.

Aripiprazole. Start with 2.5 mg or 5 mg every other day and gradually increase the dose to 7.5, 10 or 15 mg / day. Lower doses of 2.5-7.5 mg / day can sometimes already have a beneficial effect and sometimes cause fewer side effects. If you feel restless while starting aripiprazole treatment, it may help to lower the dose.

Clozapine. Start with 25 mg (or 12.5 mg) and build up very gradually. Give before sleep. Determination of the level of clozapine in the blood is necessary. For the first eighteen weeks weekly and later monthly, the white blood cells should be checked.

Flupenthixol. Start with 1 mg / day and gradually increase to a maximum of 5 mg. Watch out for acute muscle spasms, stiffness and tremors. Then at least lower the dose and temporarily give biperiden for muscle cramps.

Haloperidol. Start with 1 mg / day and gradually increase to a maximum of 5 mg. Watch out for acute muscle spasms, stiffness and tremors. Then at least reduce the dose and temporarily take biperiden in case of muscle cramps.

Lurasidone. 37 mg to 111 mg per day.

Olanzapine. Start with 5 mg / day, preferably before sleep, as olanzapine can make you sleepy. Often the optimal dose is between 5 and 20 mg per day.

Penfluridol. This antipsychotic only needs to be taken once a week. Start with 10 mg and build up to usually 20 mg.

Pimozide. Start with 1 mg / day and gradually increase to a maximum of 5 mg. Watch out for acute muscle spasms, stiffness and tremors. Then at least reduce the dose and take biperiden in case of muscle cramps.

Pipamperon. 40 mg to 160 mg per day.

Perphenazine. Start with 8 mg and increase to 16 mg / day if necessary.

Quetiapine. Start with 100 mg at night and gradually build up to 400 to 600 mg as needed.

Risperidone. Start with 1 mg per day and increase to a maximum of 5 mg. Risperidone has similar side effects to haloperidol and can also cause a significant increase in prolactin, which can cause sexual function disorders, among other things.

Sulpiride. 200 mg to 800 mg if necessary.

Zuclopenthixol. Start with 5 mg and increase to about 20 mg / day if necessary (Knegtering R and Bruggeman R. 2018).

What is meant by mg haloperidol equivalent?

Haloperidol equivalent is a general measure of the strength of an antipsychotic. Haloperidol is the standard antipsychotic for this. The dose of another antipsychotic can be converted into mg haloperidol equivalent to determine its relative potency. For example: 1 mg risperidone is as strong as 1 mg haloperidol. So, 3 mg risperidone is 3 mg haloperidol equivalent. Another example: 5 mg olanzapine is as strong as 1 mg haloperidol. So, 15 mg of olanzapine is 3 mg haloperidol equivalent. This conversion factor is less clear for some other antipsychotics. Nevertheless, an estimate can be made. For example, 150 mg of quetiapine is thought to be about as strong as 1 mg of haloperidol. So, 600 mg of quetiapine is approximately 4 mg of haloperidol equivalent.

Is there a clear difference between "old" and "new" antipsychotics?

Initially, it was thought that the new antipsychotics were better than the old ones. But that was partly because the new drugs in research were compared with too high doses of the old drugs. As a result, it seemed as if the new drugs had fewer side effects. The question of whether the old or the new antipsychotics are better was examined later. This was done by researchers who were independent of the pharmaceutical companies. In a large study in which the use of the "old" drug perphenazine was compared with, among others, the “new” drugs olanzapine, quetiapine and risperidone for a year and a half. The primary outcome measure was: how long does someone use the drug? The thought was: if someone is satisfied with the effect and experiences few side effects, then someone is inclined to continue to use the drug. Within 18 months, 64 percent of the patients taking olanzapine quit. That was significantly better than the rest: 74 percent quitted with risperidone, 75 percent with perphenazine and with quetiapine, 82 percent of the patients stopped within 18 months. It was striking that most patients therefore stopped taking the antipsychotic with which they started the study within a year and a half. Apparently, most patients do not continue to use their first antipsychotic medication. The old drug (perphenazine) did no worse than two of the new drugs (risperidone and quetiapine).

In the same way, old and new drugs were studied in patients with a first psychotic episode. Haloperidol, amisulpride, olanzapine and quetiapine were compared with each other. After a one-year follow-up, it was found that patients on a low dose of haloperidol discontinued more often than patients on a low dose of the other antipsychotics. There were no differences in the extent to which the symptoms improved.

All in all, there is no clear difference between “old” and “new” antipsychotics as a group. There are differences between certain antipsychotics in effect, but especially in side effects. More on that later.

Start of antipsychotics and acute treatment

What should you and your psychiatrist discuss before starting an antipsychotic?

Before starting an antipsychotic, you and your psychiatrist should first discuss which symptoms should be reduced by the antipsychotic. So, you agree on a goal for the treatment with the antipsychotic. This can be, for example, improving poor sleep, reducing anxiety, suspicion, hallucinations, delusions or confusion.

In addition, it is important to discuss which side effects can occur and what to do about it. Consider side effects such as dizziness, sleepiness, increased appetite, flattening of emotions, muscle cramps, difficulty sitting still and feeling restless inside, stiffness in the muscles, tremors, salivation, walking with small steps and becoming dizzy.

If you are on antipsychotics that bind strongly to the dopamine receptor, it is wise to agree on medication to take if you develop muscle cramps. This "rescue medication" could be, for example: biperiden 2 mg three times a day. Acute muscle cramps mainly occur at the beginning of treatment and especially in young men, especially after recent cocaine use. The risk of acute muscle cramps is much smaller if the dose of antipsychotics is gradually built up (Knegtering R and Bruggeman R. 2018).

When is treatment with antipsychotics not necessary for psychotic symptoms?

Whether antipsychotic treatment is needed depends on the cause, duration and severity of the psychosis, the underlying condition and a number of other factors. Here are some cases where antipsychotic treatment is not necessary in the first place:

If someone has developed a psychosis from taking street drugs and the psychotic state is not severe or dangerous, the first treatment advice is to stop street drug use and see if the psychotic symptoms disappear in the course of a few days. When the psychosis has disappeared, the advice is never to use drugs again. If the psychotic symptoms persist and are bothersome, then treatment with the lowest possible dose of antipsychotic is indicated.

If someone has developed psychotic symptoms after a traumatic experience, it is also wise to wait whether the symptoms decrease through treatment of the post-traumatic stress disorder.

If someone develops psychotic symptoms after an operation, the policy is primarily aimed at promoting the best possible function of the brain and stimulating a good day-night rhythm with sufficient rest and sufficient activity.

If someone develops a psychosis from the use of certain medication, it must first be determined whether the psychosis disappears by stopping the medication or reducing the dose.

If someone develops psychosis during depression or mania, it is wise to treat the depression or mania first. When the mood improves, the psychotic symptoms often disappear too.

If someone with an autism spectrum disorder develops psychotic symptoms in a situation in which he or she has to deal with too many stimuli, then the first treatment option is trying to reduce the amount of stimuli and strengthening the structure someone is helping someone to regain control.

If someone with a personality disorder has psychotic symptoms, then psychotherapy is the appropriate treatment in the first place.

Is antipsychotic treatment always necessary in someone with schizophrenia?

Treatment with antipsychotics is not always necessary in someone with schizophrenia. Research shows that about 13 to 20 percent of people who meet the classification criteria of schizophrenia have a psychosis only once and that they do not develop a new psychotic period. So, these people do not need maintenance treatment. At the moment we cannot predict who will belong to this group. We hope to learn more about this in the ongoing HAMLETT study. On the other hand, this also means that for 80 percent or more of the patients who meet the schizophrenia classification, antipsychotic treatment is useful in reducing the risk of a new psychotic episode.

Is treatment without antipsychotics also effective in people with schizophrenia spectrum disorder?

Certainly, there are therapeutic interventions other than antipsychotics that help reduce the severity of psychotic symptoms in people with schizophrenia spectrum disorder. You can think of stopping street drugs and reducing stress. Support from others can help, and so can an environment that feels safe and secure. Yet it is usually the case that these interventions are not sufficient to significantly reduce the severity of psychotic symptoms. Therefore, guidelines recommend treating patients to whom this applies with antipsychotics. Because antipsychotics have dose-dependent side effects, because the dopamine system should not be overly inhibited and because too high a dose is not more effective, the lowest possible effective dose should be sought.

There are small-scale initiatives that attempt to use little or no antipsychotics. These are the so-called Soteria projects.

What is the history of the Soteria project?

In the 1970s, a small-scale experimental setting was established near San Francisco to treat young patients with schizophrenia with psychotherapy and environmental therapy methods, and with a minimum of medication. The emphasis was on the therapeutic power of the relationship, the reason why there was a restful other person around the patient all the time, and a safe home environment. There were positive expectations for recovery. In addition, much attention was paid to the value of the subjective psychotic experience. Patients retained personal freedom of decision and were involved in household chores. If psychotic symptoms did not worsen or started to improve during the first six weeks, no antipsychotics were prescribed. If psychotic symptoms persisted after six weeks, the lowest effective dose was given.

A similar project was started near Bern in Switzerland in the 1980s. Based on the idea that psychosis develops with emotional tension, an attempt was made to create an environment with as little stress as possible. If psychotic symptoms did not resolve within a few days, antipsychotics were started. Soteria houses have since been established in Germany, Hungary, Israel and the Netherlands. An international organization, the Soteria-Netzwerk, was created (see www.soteria-netzwerk.de). It is emphasized that at least five years aftercare is required.

Are there any data on the efficacy of Soteria care?

Calton wrote a systematic review article on the effectiveness of Soteria care. Three controlled studies have been performed. One study was randomized, in one study patients were placed alternately in the Soteria house or in a regular ward, and in the last study patients were placed in a regular psychiatric ward when there was no room in the Soteria house. The latter two ways of distributing patients over the different treatment forms are methodologically weak, because they increase the likelihood of an unequal distribution of confounding factors influencing the outcome.

Before interpreting the outcomes of Soteria care, it is important to realize that Soteria care is not dogmatic anti-medication. About 24 percent of patients who received Soteria care received antipsychotics in the first six weeks of treatment, and 57 percent of them were on antipsychotics after two years. In the group of patients who received regular treatment, this was 100 percent in the first six weeks and 97 percent after two years. In another study, 73 percent of Soteria patients were on antipsychotics after two years, versus 95 percent of patients on regular treatment. The results of these three studies did not show any major differences in outcome between the Soteria and the regular treatment. Long-term outcome data is lacking. In addition, these studies were conducted at a time when it was common practice in routine treatment to prescribe antipsychotics in high doses. The founder of the Bern house, Luc Ciompi, described that the average length of stay has decreased over the years from 185 days to 44 days. About 10 to 15 percent of patients cannot be treated in this open setting because of the lack of collaboration. In less than 1 percent of treatments serious incidents were reported, but Ciompi did not describe what these were. Ciompi emphasized that a Soteria house must be attached to a psychiatric hospital, as admission to a closed ward is sometimes required.

I think these studies confirm that it is worth treating with the lowest possible dose, but I do not believe that treatment without antipsychotics offers an equally good alternative for most patients.

What physical examination should be done before starting antipsychotics?

Before starting antipsychotics, your medical history and current physical symptoms should be discussed. In addition, heart rate, blood pressure, height, weight and waist circumference must be measured.

Which laboratory tests should be carried out, preferably before you start taking antipsychotics?

Before you start taking antipsychotics, a few things are preferably examined in a laboratory: the sedimentation speed of the red blood cells (this says something about possible inflammation), white blood cells, enzymes that say something about your liver function, electrolytes that say something about your kidney function, blood sugar (preferably fasting), cholesterol and triglycerides. Sometimes it is not possible to do these tests before starting an antipsychotic (Knegtering R and Bruggeman R. 2018).

How high should the dosage of an antipsychotic be?

The dose required to reduce psychosis varies from person to person. The dosage that causes side effects also varies from person to person. The required dosage depends, among other things, on the speed with which someone breaks down and excrete the antipsychotic. In many adults, 2 to 4 mg haloperidol equivalents per day appears to be sufficient. Whether you have for the first time in your life a psychotic episode or whether you have had more episodes and antipsychotic treatment is also important. People who have a psychotic episode for the first time are more sensitive to antipsychotics. They need lower doses, around 2 mg haloperidol equivalents. If extrapyramidal side effects occur (see later in this chapter), too many dopamine receptors are occupied and the dose should be reduced. Not everyone's psychotic symptoms disappear completely. When being treated with antipsychotics, you should strive for optimal relief of symptoms with as few side effects as possible. Higher doses than needed to occupy about 70% of the dopaminereceptors are not more effective, while the risk of side effects increases (Knegtering R and Bruggeman R. 2018).

Why is it that the optimal dosage of an antipsychotic can differ so much from person to person?

The fact that the optimal dosage of an antipsychotic can differ from person to person is partly due to genetic differences between people in the rate at which the antipsychotic is broken down in the liver. As a result, the same dose produces a lower blood level in one person than in another. It may also be due to a genetic difference in the speed at which an antipsychotic crosses the blood-brain barrier surrounding the brain. In addition, the dopamine system also differs substantially between people. As earlier mentioned, it is also often the case that a lower dose is required for a first psychosis than for a second psychosis.

It is difficult to predict the effect of drugs for an individual. That is annoying, but you have to try and find out which antipsychotic in which dosage is best for you.

How quickly do you notice the antipsychotic effect of antipsychotics?

How soon you notice the antipsychotic effect of antipsychotics also differs per person, but usually the effect is noticeable quickly. In general, after one or two weeks of treatment, an assessment is made to see whether the medication is effective. If no effect occurs after two weeks, the chance is very small that this will happen in the future. It may also be that the dosage is too low. Or that you did not use it as prescribed. Or that you continued to use street-drugs. If there are no dose-dependent side effects, the dose can be further increased cautiously.

When should you assess the effect of an antipsychotic?

You normally assess the effect of an antipsychotic after one or two weeks, but at least after four weeks. (With clozapine it may take longer for a beneficial effect to become noticeable and the effect may also gradually increase in the weeks to months thereafter) A good effect during the first few days is a predictor of a good effect in the long term. If there is no good effect after two to four weeks, it can be checked in the blood whether the level of the antipsychotic drug is perhaps too low. This could be because someone breaks down and excretes the antipsychotic quickly. If someone does not recover at all after two to four weeks, with a good dose and good adherence, it is wise to choose another antipsychotic with a different receptor binding profile. If someone does not recover from this either, then you speak of therapy resistance. Thereafter treatment with clozapine is indicated.

It is common for some psychotic symptoms to remain partially present. Increasing the dosage further is often not useful. In a not insignificant proportion of people, the psychotic symptoms do not completely diminish during treatment with antipsychotics. Then it is wise to find an optimal dose with a reasonable effect and as few unwanted effects as possible.

Does it make sense to determine the blood level of an antipsychotic?

For haloperidol and clozapine an association between blood levels and effect has been shown. This relationship is unclear for many other antipsychotics. Sometimes it can be useful to measure a blood level to find out if someone has taken an antipsychotic or to check the blood level. In addition to the dose, the blood level also depends on the speed at which someone breaks down the antipsychotic.

Antipsychotics to prevent a relapse of psychosis

How should you take antipsychotics to prevent a recurrence of psychosis?

Antipsychotics reduce psychotic symptoms, but do not cure vulnerability. Most people would like to stop taking antipsychotics when the psychosis is over.

Understandably, you'd rather go without pills. Yet in a considerable number of cases that is not wise. If you stop taking antipsychotics, the psychosis may come back. If your condition meets the classification schizophrenia, there is about an 80 percent chance that the psychosis will come back in the course of two years when you stop taking antipsychotics. Continuing to take antipsychotics reduces that chance to about 20 percent. The risk of a recurrence of the psychosis also depends on your history. If you have already had two psychotic periods in your life, the chance of a new psychosis after stopping treatment with antipsychotics is even greater than 80 percent. That is why it is advised to keep taking antipsychotics if you have had multiple psychoses. Always look for the lowest effective dose.

How high is the optimal dose during maintenance treatment?

In the past, it was recommended to give about 50 to 60 percent of the dose needed to treat the acute psychosis during maintenance treatment. However, since very low doses are often already given today during the acute treatment of psychosis, it is sometimes wiser not to go below about 75 percent of that dose. So, if you have recovered from 10 mg olanzapine, it is recommended that you use no less than 7.5 mg in the maintenance treatment. But it may be safer to continue the use of 10 mg. Even if you recovered from 20 mg olanzapine, it is likely that a maintenance dose should not fall below 15 mg. From studies in patients with multiple episodes it appeared that the dosage should be at least 3.5 mg HE. The dosage should always be tapered very gradually over months. However, it sometimes remains a difficult decision. After all, too high a maintenance dose increases the risk of undesirable effects, such as a flattening of the emotional life and less energy and motivation. On the other hand, dosages that are too low increase the risk of a recurrence of psychosis, with the associated adverse consequences.

Because you are in a calmer phase after the acute psychosis, there is room to look for the optimal dose together with your professional caregiver. The difficult thing is that a new psychosis usually does not develop immediately after dose reduction. It sometimes takes a long time, sometimes even months, before another psychosis occurs. So, you only know after a while whether you are "right" with your lower dose. Therefore, it is wise to lower the antipsychotic dose a little and then wait quite some time (several months) before trying any further reduction. It is not recommended to reduce the dosage on your own (Knegtering R and Bruggeman R. 2018).

When is maintenance treatment useful and how long should it last?

Many guidelines recommend continuing the use of antipsychotics for one to two years in the treatment of schizophrenia after a first psychosis. If there have been multiple psychotic episodes, continuous maintenance treatment is recommended. Temporary treatment and attempts to quit clearly increase the risk of a new psychosis.

Although it is clear that antipsychotics significantly reduce the risk of new psychosis, they do not always improve social functioning. For this reason, there is currently uncertainty about the treatment of patients who have recovered from a first psychosis. Who can better receive longer-term maintenance treatment and who can gradually reduce its use? To get more clarity about this, the HAMLETT study has been started. The results of this study will become available after 2025.

Based on a comparable study, Lex Wunderink believes that an attempt to gradual reduce antipsychotics may be justified if a number of conditions are met: - Patients do not experience bothersome psychotic symptoms anymore. - The patient and his family members are and will remain involved in the treatment. -There is close contact with the professional caregiver, so that help is available quickly if there are signs of a new psychosis. -The patient realizes that the chance of a new psychosis with gradual withdrawal is at least two times larger in the first year.

What are the chances that someone who meets the criteria for schizophrenia and has fully recovered from a first psychosis will be able to successfully stop taking antipsychotics?

About one in five patients who meet the schizophrenia classification and who have fully recovered from a first psychosis can successfully stop taking antipsychotics. The problem is, we don't know in advance who can stop. We hope to learn more about this through the HAMLETT study.

What is an Antipsychotic Depot?

A depot is a way to administrate an antipsychotic. Via an injection into a large muscle in your body (usually your buttock muscle), an amount of an antipsychotic in liquid form is injected. This antipsychotic enters the bloodstream very gradually over the following weeks, and from there moves into the brain. The speed at which this happens differs per depot. Some depots are sufficient for one month, some are sufficient for two weeks.

Are there any antipsychotics that you can take orally that work for more than a day?

Penfluridol works for about seven days, which means you only need to take a pill once a week.

What can be the benefits of an antipsychotic in depot form?

If it is difficult to take pills regularly, a depot can be a solution. Research of registers in which medication and admissions are kept shows that people with the classification schizophrenia who use a depot are less likely to be readmitted than people who take antipsychotics orally.

Therapy resistance

What is the definition of therapy resistance?

If there is insufficient effect of two consecutive adequate antipsychotic treatments, this is referred to as therapy resistance. By adequate treatment is meant: the antipsychotic is taken, the dose was high enough and it has been tried long enough (about four weeks per antipsychotic). Therapy resistance therefore means that the usual therapy does not work. If there is therapy resistance, it is wise to try treatment with clozapine.

What effect does clozapine have in patients with treatment resistance?

About 50 percent of patients who failed to respond to two other antipsychotics still experience a beneficial effect of clozapine on psychotic symptoms.

Why is clozapine not used as a first-choice medicine?

Clozapine is not used as a first choice because its side effects can be severe and can have serious consequences. In about 1 percent of patients on clozapine, a decrease in white blood cells may occur, which means that infections are no longer effectively controlled. If the white blood cell count becomes too low, clozapine treatment should be discontinued. Therefore, regular monitoring of the white blood cell count is needed. Furthermore, people are often sleepy (especially at the beginning of treatment) and dizzy when getting up (because the blood pressure does not rise quickly enough), they may suffer from salivation and constipation, substantial weight gain is common and there is a small chance of heart disease. Not all patients are eligible for treatment with clozapine, as compliance with blood monitoring and careful use must be ensured.

Differences between Antipsychotics

Are there differences in effectiveness on psychotic symptoms between antipsychotics?

On the basis of meta-analyzes it is possible to make a ranking of effectiveness. In general, there are no large group differences in effectiveness between the various antipsychotics.

I used meta-analyzes, randomized studies and research into receptor occupancy by antipsychotics to create a ranking of antipsychotics. Based on these findings, I made rankings for different aspects of effectiveness and for different side effects. The ranking for "Effectiveness on global severity of psychotic symptoms" is shown in Table 41.1.

Table 41.1 Effectiveness on global severity of psychotic symptoms

clozapine -0.89
amisulpride -0.73
olanzapine -0.56
perphenazine -0.56
risperidone -0.55
zuclopenthixol -0.51
sulpiride -0.48
haloperidol -0.47
quetiapine -0.42
aripiprazole -0.41
penfluridol -0.39
lurasidone -0.36
cariprazine -0.34
pimozide -0.30
brexpiprazole -0.26
flupentixol -0.24

The number that you see behind the antipsychotics is the effect size compared to placebo. You can see that clozapine has the greatest effect (-0.89) followed by amisulpride (-0.73) and olanzapine (-0.56).

You should also take into account that the differences as shown in the table are based on the mean difference between groups. It can work out differently for individuals. Aripiprazole may very well be more effective for you than olanzapine. The ranking provides an estimate of the chances of difference in effectiveness (or side effects) in groups (Van Dijk F, et al. 2018).

Are there differences in effectiveness on depressive symptoms between antipsychotics?

In the same way as described in the above question, I also ranked the effectiveness of antipsychotics on depressive symptoms. However, a warning is in order here: effectiveness on depressive symptoms is almost never the primary outcome measure of antipsychotic research. In addition, there are also have less data on effectiveness on depressive symptoms. With these limitations in mind, see the ranking shown in Table 41.2. The number behind the antipsychotic is the effect size compared to placebo (Van Dijk F, et al. 2018).

Table 41.2 Effectiveness on depressive symptoms

sulpiride –0.90
clozapine -0.52
amisulpride -0.44
aripiprazole -0.40
olanzapine -0.37
cariprazine -0.36
quetiapine -0.24
risperidone -0.23
lurasidone -0.20
pimozide -0.20
penfluridol -0.18
haloperidol -0.17
zuclopentixol-0.16
flupenthixol 0.04

Are there differences in effectiveness on attention and memory between antipsychotics?

In general, antipsychotics have a beneficial effect on attention and memory in people with psychosis. This is certainly also related to the dosage of antipsychotics. Too high doses can impair attention (and probably therefore also memory). However, little research has been done into the difference in the effect of antipsychotics on attention and memory. Therefore, the findings are not very robust.

Do some antipsychotics have a more beneficial effect on negative symptoms?

There is limited evidence that amisulpride, clozapine and olanzapine have a slightly more beneficial effect on negative symptoms compared to the other antipsychotics. Because the differences are very small and uncertain, I decided not to rank antipsychotics on this criterium.

On average, antipsychotics have a beneficial effect on negative symptoms. This is probably because negative symptoms (eg withdrawal behavior) are associated with the severity of psychotic symptoms. When people become less suspicious during treatment with antipsychotics, it is easier to get among people again. However, higher doses can sometimes aggravate negative symptoms. Even at average doses, there is sometimes more fatigue, dullness, depression and withdrawal and a greater lack of initiative. These adverse effects require adjustment of antipsychotic treatment.

Do the side effects differ per antipsychotic?

Are there differences in side effects between antipsychotics?

The differences in side effects between antipsychotics are more substantial than the differences in effect. That is why it is good that there are many different types of antipsychotics, although unfortunately we cannot determine in advance which one will work best for whom. Side effects can be related to too high a dosage, but also to specific properties of the antipsychotic. Side effects can occur, for example, if an antipsychotic also affects receptors other than the dopamine receptor.

What other receptors are affected by some antipsychotics?

Some antipsychotics such as clozapine and olanzapine affect other receptors in addition to dopamine receptors, such as serotonin, noradrenergic, histamine, muscarinic and cholinergic receptors. This affects the effect and side effects. More about that in the below.

What could be the result of a potent inhibitory effect on cholinergic receptors?

Clozapine and olanzapine have a strong anticholinergic effect. This can help reduce the risk of parkinsonism or acute dystonia, but it can also exacerbate memory problems and even can cause confusion in the elderly. Dry mouth, increased pressure in the eyes, more difficult urination and delayed bowel movements can also be caused by anticholinergic effects.

What could be the result of a potent inhibitory effect on histaminergic receptors?

Clozapine, olanzapine and quetiapine strongly block the histamine receptor. This increases the risk of drowsiness and weight gain.

What could be the result of a potent inhibitory effect on noradrenergic receptors?

Clozapine and quetiapine strongly block noradrenergic receptors. This is thought to have antidepressant effects, but it can also cause dizziness when standing up and less sex drive. A rare but potentially dangerous side effect is the development of a long-lasting erection. If this continues for several hours, the blood supply to the penis may be compromised. This is an acute emergency. Patients are often embarrassed about this, but if it occurs, medical help should be sought quickly!!

What effect can antipsychotics have on subjective experience?

About 30% of the people experience a flattening of emotional life when taking antipsychotics: they experience fewer feelings of pleasure and sadness. Unpleasant subjective effects of antipsychotics can be an important reason to stop taking medication. It is important to note that about 70 percent of patients actually have an improved subjective experience after starting treatment with antipsychotics.

The subjective experience with an antipsychotic appears to depend mainly on the dosage and occupation of dopamine receptors. The occupancy of dopamine receptors with the same amount of antipsychotic may differ from patient to patient. That is why adjusting someone to the correct dosage is tailor-made.

How do you choose an antipsychotic that does not have unacceptable side effects?

Because the risks of side effects differ per antipsychotic, you really have something to choose. Some antipsychotics increase the risk of weight gain, other antipsychotics increase the risk of muscle tremors or stiffness. That is why side effects are often a reason to switch to a different antipsychotic. However, the degree to which a side effect is undesirable could also be a factor in the decision to start with a particular antipsychotic or not.

Below I discuss various side effects of antipsychotics. You will find a ranking per side effect. These rankings are based on scientific research into how often an adverse reaction occurs compared to treatment with placebo or other antipsychotics. The antipsychotics higher in the ranking are associated with a greater risk of this side effect. Sometimes there is no research into a particular side effect with a particular antipsychotic. In that case, an estimate is made of the risk of side effects for that antipsychotic on the basis of receptor profiles and other characteristics of an antipsychotic.

It is important to realize that this information intended as a decision aid: the outcome does not guarantee that an antipsychotic is effective for you or that side effects will not occur. This also applies to the rankings below. Everyone reacts differently to a drug. Your professional caregiver can also have good reasons for an opinion that differs from the result of the ranking. In addition, switching antipsychotics can also cause problems. Sometimes new antipsychotics work less well and the old antipsychotic also works less well when you return to them. That is why it is wise to switch only if there are clear advantages to be expected. It is advisable to discuss this with each other and to come to a choice together. In short: it goes without saying that you can decide together to choose a different antipsychotic than the one listed here. If you have already had good experiences with an antipsychotic, keep using these. Never change a winning team.

Does one antipsychotic cause weight gain more often than another?

There is considerable evidence that some antipsychotics lead to more weight gain than others. This may be because some stimulate the appetite and/or inhibit the feeling of satiety, causing you to eat more than is good for you. Especially clozapine and olanzapine, but also other new antipsychotics such as quetiapine and risperidone cause on average considerable weight gain compared to the alternatives. The figure in Table 41.4 behind the antipsychotic is the effect size relative to placebo (Van Dijk F, et al. 2018).

Table 41.4 Probability of weight gain

clozapine 3.01
olanzapine 2.73
quetiapine 1.56
risperidone 1.28
brexpiprazole 0.88
flupentixol 0.75
cariprazine 0.66
amisulpride 0.66
zuclopentixol 0.53
sulpiride 0.53
aripiprazole 0.34
lurasidone 0.32
haloperidol 0.23
pimozide no evidence to rank this antipsychotic
perphenazine no evidence to rank this antipsychotic
penfluridol no evidence to rank this antipsychotic
pipamperone no evidence to rank this antipsychotic

Is one antipsychotic more likely to cause sexual function problems than another?

Risperidone and its derivative paliperidone cause sexual dysfunction much more often than the other antipsychotics. Blocking dopamine in combination with an increase in the amount of prolactin in the blood appears to be an important underlying mechanism. Risperidone and paliperidone have a breakdown product that does not enter the brain itself, but does block dopamine receptors outside the brain. As a result, the blockade of dopamine receptors in the pituitary gland becomes high, and this causes prolactin to rise sharply. A high prolactin level is associated with breast enlargement (also in men), milk flow from the nipples (can also occur in men), erectile dysfunction, menstrual disorders and less sex drive. These side effects are not permanent, they disappear when the drug is discontinued or the dosage is reduced. The other antipsychotics that potently occupy the dopamine receptor are also associated with dose-dependent prolactin elevation and associated sexual dysfunction. The least prolactin increase is found with the antipsychotics that bind loosely (clozapine and quetiapine) or with aripiprazole, because the latter both inhibits and stimulates dopamine.

The figure that you see behind the antipsychotic in Table 41.5 is the effect size on the prolactin level compared to placebo. You can see that amisulpiride, sulpiride and risperidone has a major effect, that is, it clearly causes more sexual function disorders than placebo. For a number of antipsychotics a minus sign represents the effect size. This means that in research they gave on average less sexual function disorders than placebo (Van Dijk F, et al. 2018).

Table 41.5 Probability of sexual function problems

amisulpride 1.38
sulpiride
risperidone 1.17
haloperidol 0.71
perphenazine
pipamperone
zuclopentixol
pimozide
penfluridol
flupentixol 0.5
lurasidone 0.28
olanzapine 0.15

brexpiprazole 0.13
cariprazine -0.1
quetiapine -0.13
aripiprazole -0.22
clozapine -2.05

Does one antipsychotic cause drowsiness more often than another?

Table 41.6 lists the probability that an antipsychotic will cause drowsiness. The relative risk [RR] is given. For instance, with clozapine 3 times as much patients experience drowsiness than with placebo (Van Dijk F, et al. 2018).

Table 41.6 Probability of drowsiness

zuclopentixol RR 10.20
sulpiride RR 4.08
quetiapine RR 3.27
clozapine RR 3.02
olanzapine RR 2.17
risperidone RR 2.03
haloperidol RR 1.92
lurasidone RR 1.75
brexpiprazole RR 1.64
amisulpride RR 1.56
aripiprazole RR 1.46
penfluridol RR 1.24
flupentixol RR 1.12
cariprazine RR 1.12
perphenazine RR 1.09
pimozide RR 0.92
pipamperone no RR

What are extrapyramidal side effects?

Extrapyramidal side effects are problems of posture or movement caused by the influence of antipsychotics. Examples of extrapyramidal side effects are less spontaneous movement, slower start of a movement, increased muscle tension and stiffness, a bent posture, the contraction of muscle groups and tremors. Parkinsonism is one of the extrapyramidal side effects.

Does one antipsychotic cause extrapyramidal side effects more often than another?

There are important differences between antipsychotics in their likelihood of causing extrapyramidal side effects. Extrapyramidal side effects occur when more than 80 percent of dopamine receptors are occupied by an antipsychotic. Whether the side effects occur depends on the dosage. Antipsychotics that bind vigorously to the dopamine receptor are most likely to cause these side effects. In Table 41.7 below, the antipsychotics are ranked based on the likelihood of extrapyramidal adverse events compared to placebo treatment. If the RR is 1, then the risk of these side effects with the drug is the same as with a placebo. If the RR is 5.14 then side effects are more than 5 times more frequent with pimozide than with placebo. And if the RR is 0.46 (as with clozapine) extrapyramidal side effects occur about 2 times as often with placebo. With other words the risk on extrapyramidal side effects with clozapine is very low (Van Dijk F, et al. 2018).

Table 41.7 Risk of extrapyramidal adverse effects

pimozide RR 5.14
flupentixol RR 3.9
penfluridol RR 3.48
haloperidol RR 3.13
zuclopentixol RR 3.06
perphenazine RR 2.64
sulpiride RR 2.38.
cariprazine RR 2.21
lurasidone RR 1.94
risperidone RR 1.80
brexpiprazole RR 1.60
amisulpride RR 1.46
aripiprazole RR 1.32
quetiapine RR 1.05
olanzapine RR 1.02
clozapine RR 0.46

What Are Anticholinergic Side Effects?

Anticholinergic side effects arise because a drug blocks choline receptors. Anticholinergic side effects include blurred vision, dry mouth, constipation, difficult urination, and decreased attention and memory. Confusion can even occur in the elderly.

Does one antipsychotic cause more anticholinergic side effects than another?

Little research has been conducted into the risk of anticholinergic side effects of antipsychotics. In Table 41.8 you can see the Relative Risk compared to placebo that anticholinergic side effects will occur (Van Dijk F, et al. 2018).

Table 41.8 Risk of anticholinergic adverse reactions

quetiapine RR 3.89
zuclopentixol RR 2.73
clozapine RR 2.21
flupentixol RR 2.14
olanzapine RR 1.94
penfluridol RR 1.63
amisulpride RR 1.53
haloperidol RR 1.50
cariprazine RR 1.45
perphenazine RR 1.32
risperidone RR 1.31
aripiprazole RR 1.30
pimozide RR 1.17
lurasidone RR 1.14
sulpiride RR 1.01
brexpiprazole RR 0.72
pipamperone no RR aivailable

Does one antipsychotic cause more salivation than another?

With salivation you produce more saliva or you swallow your saliva less quickly, so that you get a wet pillow at night. Table 41.9 shows the average percentage of patients who have (some) problems with salivation when they use that antipsychotic (Van Dijk F, et al. 2018).

Table 41.9 Risk of salivation

clozapine 32.7%
zuclopenthixol 24.2%
haloperidol 18.4%
olanzapine 8.2%
amisulpride 7.8%
risperidone 5.7%
penfluridol no evidence
flupentixol no evidence
aripiprazole no evidence
lurasidone no evidence
sulpiride no evidence
perphenazine no evidence
pipamperon no evidence
quetiapine no evidence
pimozide no evidence

Is one antipsychotic more likely to cause dizziness than another?

The risk of dizziness when standing up depends on the effect of antipsychotics on the so-called alpha 1 receptor. Table 41.11 has been drawn up on the basis of the extent to which antipsychotics bind to this receptor. The lower the α1-receptor affinity the higher the binding to this receptor and the higher the risk of dizziness. Be aware that this ranking is not based on research in patients but on the the α1-receptor affinity (Van Dijk F, et al. 2018).

Table 41.11 Risk of dizziness

clozapine	α1-receptor affinity 1.6
risperidone	α1-receptor affinity 5
perphenazine	α1-receptor affinity 10
haloperidol	α1-receptor affinity 12
quetiapine	α1-receptor affinity 22
brexpiprazole	α1-receptor affinity 24
aripiprazole	α1-receptor affinity 25
lurasidone	α1-receptor affinity 47
pipamperone	α1-receptor affinity 66
olanzapine	A1-receptor affinity 109
pimozide	α1-receptor affinity 138
cariprazine	α1-receptor affinity > 379

amisulpride	α1-receptor affinity > 10,000
sulpiride	α1-receptor affinity > 10,000
penfluridol	No data available
flupentixol	No data available
zuclopentixol	No data available

Is one antipsychotic more likely to cause fatigue than another?

Only one study has been conducted into antipsychotic fatigue, so very little is known about the differences between various drugs. One study found that people taking aripiprazole were less tired than people taking other antipsychotics. I decided to mention this despite the lack of research, because it is also understandable from the mechanism of action that aripiprazole is less likely to cause fatigue: aripiprazole also stimulates the dopamine system (Van Dijk F, et al. 2018).

Is one antipsychotic more likely to cause a feeling of inhibition than another?

The dampening effect of antipsychotics does not only affect experiences and thoughts that are given too much importance. Especially when the dosage of an antipsychotic is too high, all thoughts and experiences become less important. Then patients complain of flattening or an unpleasant feeling of numbness while taking antipsychotics. This unpleasant feeling indicates that the effect of dopamine is too much inhibited. Then it is wise to look for a lower dose or an antipsychotic that attaches less strongly to the dopamine receptor together with your professional caregiver. The sensitivity to this side effect of antipsychotics is related to individual characteristics of the dopamine system. That is why customization is needed.

The sense of flattening is the flip side of the fundamental mechanism of antipsychotics: dampening the importance you place on impressions or thoughts. After all, this is the driving force behind our activities and interactions. It is likely that the same mechanism that takes the fire out of symptoms can also dampen normal motivation and desires, pleasure and meaningful experiences. Therefore, the lowest possible effective dose should always be sought in the treatment of psychosis. Enough to have less problems with delusions, hallucinations and confusion, but at the same time not too much, so that motivation is hardly or not at all hindered by it. Too much dampening can result from too high a dose of an antipsychotic that attaches vigorously to the dopamine receptor. With antipsychotics that bind less strongly to the dopamine receptor, this feeling of inhibition and dampening is less common. In addition, it occurs less with aripiprazole, cariprazine and brexpiprazole because these agents have an inhibitory as well as an excitatory effect on dopamine (Van Dijk F, et al. 2018).

Table 41.13 Chance of feeling inhibited

perphenazine	D2 affinity 1
lurasidone	D2 affinity 1.7
haloperidol	D2 affinity 2
zuclopenthixol	D2 affinity 2
amisulpride	D2 affinity 2,4
risperidon	D2 affinity 4.9
penfluridol	D2 affinity 5.6
pimozide	D2 affinity 6
pipamperone	D2 affinity 7
sulpiride	D2 affinity
olanzapine	D2 affinity 72
clozapine	D2 affinity 431
quetiapine	D2 affinity 567
cariprazine	partial agonism
brexpiprazole	partial agonism
aripiprazole	partial agonism

Does one antipsychotic cause seizures more often than another?

Table 41.14 shows a percentage behind the antipsychotic. For example, a percentage of 9 percent means that 9 percent of the serious side effects of that antipsychotic involved an epileptic seizure. That's a bit of a weird way of sorting out the risk of this side effect, but it was the only information I could find. Seizures caused by an antipsychotic are rare. You should especially consider the risk of this side effect when you have previously had an epileptic seizure. The table 41.14 is complicated. The number 9% means that an epileptic seizure accounted for 9% of the serious side effects. So not in 9% of the patients! The same applies to the other percentages mentioned (Van Dijk F, et al. 2018).

Table 41.14 Percentage of serious side effects being an epileptic seizure

clozapine 9.0%
quetiapine 5.9%
olanzapine 4.9%
zuclopenthixol 4.2%

risperidone 3.7%
pimozide 3.4%
haloperidol 3.3%
perphenazine 3.2%
flupentixol 2.6%
aripiprazole 2.6%
sulpiride 0.5%

Could it make sense to add other medications to antipsychotics?

If treatment with clozapine does not help, does it make sense to add other medications?

In review articles of placebo-controlled double-blind studies, no convincingly effective strategies are found, mainly due to the small number of studies, which moreover often contradict each other. Nevertheless, there are two drugs that have been studied in addition to antipsychotics in at least 400 patients in studies of fairly good quality and that have a reasonable effect size. These are estrogens and topiramate. Estrogens had an effect size of -0.38 on positive symptoms compared to the addition of placebo. And topiramate had an effect size of -0.37 on positive symptoms compared to the addition of placebo.

Does adding memantine to clozapine help reduce negative symptoms?

A number of studies indicate that adding 20 mg of memantine per day to clozapine may produce a limited reduction in negative symptoms and also some improvement in cognitive symptoms.

Does adding antidepressants to antipsychotics help reduce negative symptoms?

Meta-analysis shows that antidepressants added to antipsychotics can reduce the severity of negative symptoms and the severity of depressive symptoms to a limited extent.

Does adding another antipsychotic to the antipsychotic you use help?

Earlier, psychiatrists thought that it was not wise to use two different antipsychotics. However, in register studies it was found that patients who used two antipsychotics were less often readmitted. That has changed the opinion of many psychiatrists.

Moreover, there are favorable reports concerning adding low-dose aripiprazole to clozapine treatment. Patients who used this combination experienced less severe negative symptoms, reduced weight gain and a smaller risk to develop obsessive compulsive symptoms in response to clozapine treatment. Therefore, in our department we always propose patients to combine clozapine treatment with low-dose aripirazole.

References

Knegtering R and Bruggeman R. 2018. "Farmacotherapie" In Handboek schizofreniespectrumstoornissen, edited by Wiepke Cahn, Inez Myin-Germeys, Richard Bruggeman, Lieuwe de Haan. Amsterdam: De Tijdstroom.

Knegtering R and Bruggeman R. 2018. "Farmacotherapie in de klinische praktijk" In Handboek schizofreniespectrumstoornissen, edited by Wiepke Cahn, Inez Myin-Germeys, Richard Bruggeman, Lieuwe de Haan. Amsterdam: De Tijdstroom.

Van Dijk F, et al. The Personal Antipsychotic Choice Index. Pharmacopsychiatry. 2018 May;51(3):89-99.

CHAPTER 42

PSYCHOTHERAPY

What is the history of psychotherapy of schizophrenia?

Emil Kraepelin (1856-1926) saw schizophrenia as a degenerative disease, and according to him psychotherapy was pointless. Eugen Bleuler (1857-1939) thought otherwise. He hypothesized that psychotherapy could help reduce the effects of a psychotic illness. Psychoanalysts came up with different theories about schizophrenia, but patients with schizophrenia were considered unsuitable for psychoanalysis. One speculative psychoanalytic idea was that delusion was a defense mechanism against depressive thoughts and suicidality. It was therefore thought that it was better not to discuss the content of delusions with patients.

Another (horrible) theory devised by a psychoanalyst was that a schizophrenogenic mother raised the child with double messages, so the child could never get it right and thus developed schizophrenia. This idea was very wrong and has made many mothers deeply unhappy.

In the 1990s, more and more attention was paid to cognitive behavioral therapy. From that moment on, the history of psychotherapy in schizophrenia becomes more favorable (Van der Gaag M et al., 2018).

What is Cognitive Therapy?

Cognitive therapy examines the relationship between thoughts and emotions. The basic idea is that negative thoughts make you anxious or depressed. The opposite is equally true: fearful feelings give you dark thoughts. In cognitive therapy, the patient and therapist examine whether the thoughts are correct and whether there may be a way of thinking that is more appropriate. In the search for more realistic and positive thoughts, homework is used, among other things.

What is Behavioral Therapy?

Behavioral therapy focuses on changing behavior. Your behavior has a major influence on how you feel and vice versa. For example, when you are afraid of something, you tend to avoid that situation. You feel less anxious in the short term. But in the long term, this limits your freedom of movement and you become more afraid, because you increasingly dread the situation you are avoiding. As a result, you become increasingly convinced that you are rightly avoiding the fearful situation. The fear of what you want to avoid increases all the time.

In behavioral therapy, the patient and the therapist together examine the problematic behavior and the circumstances in which the behavior occurs. Then they look for more appropriate behavioral patterns in those circumstances. You will practice this in real life. During a severe phase of a psychosis, this practice is often difficult, but becoming active and challenge your fears may be possible after a while.

What is Cognitive Behavioral Therapy?

Cognitive behavioral therapy is a combination of the two forms of psychotherapy mentioned above. Cognitive behavioral therapy assumes that a person's thoughts and behavior influence the development and persistence of problems. By examining and changing thoughts and behavior, problems can be alleviated. It is a treatment that expects action from the patient. You will be given homework assignments to practice outside of the conversations. Cognitive behavioral therapy has been extensively researched and appears to be an effective psychotherapy with limited beneficial effects.

How are delusions dealt with in cognitive behavioral therapy?

A delusion is seen as an attempt to understand and explain experiences and events. But it is an attempt that causes problems: you or others are bothered by it. In cognitive behavioral therapy, you and your therapist will investigate whether the delusion is really correct. You are encouraged to think about the evidence for the delusion. If you manage to doubt it a bit, you can test the delusion in a behavioral experiment.

Suppose you believe that everyone can read your mind, then a behavioral experiment could be that you think of a certain number below hundred and that someone else gets ten dollars from you if she guesses that number. The chance that someone will succeed in this is one in a hundred, so this experiment can easily make you doubt. You can try to agree that you get ten dollars if they don't guess. That is an easy way to become rich. And you get proof that people cannot read your mind.

In the cognitive-behavioral treatment of suspicious delusions, attention is paid to your tendency to be especially aware of danger. By avoiding what is believed to be a dangerous situation, your belief in the delusion remains. If you think that others will attack you when you go out and you therefore always stay indoors, you can never experience that it is not so bad outside. Exposing yourself to the presumed danger is an important part of the treatment.

Your tendency to jump to conclusions is also addressed in the treatment and you are encouraged to come up with multiple explanations for the things that have happened to you (Van der Gaag M et al., 2018).

How is it that avoiding scary situations makes suspicion persist?

Avoidance keeps anxious expectations untested. As a result, you don't learn that certain actions can be safe and reassuring and paranoid thoughts persist (or even get stronger over time). It can help if you notice that your greatest fear is not coming true. But during a psychosis it is often not easy at all. Then it seems that there is always a sign that will keep you convinced that your thoughts are true after all. For instance: You can see from the way people look that they have malicious plans. If things are not too bad for a moment, then that is nice for that moment, but the next day the suspicion can return. Beliefs can be tough. This is partly because we humans are inclined to always perceive things that fit our beliefs. It is difficult to look critically and with a fresh look.

How is avoidance dealt with in cognitive behavioral therapy?

In cognitive-behavioral therapy, people learn to conduct behavioral experiments in the social environment, in order to actively test their negative expectations. If they find out that their negative expectations are not being fulfilled, they will adjust these thoughts a bit and the suspicion may subside.

How does cognitive behavioral therapy deal with hearing voices?

Cognitive behavioral therapy for voices focuses on the beliefs you have about the origin, power and purpose of the voices. The beliefs about the voices are explored with the therapist through previous events and behavioral experiments. Suppose you hear a voice giving you commands and suppose that voice says that if you do not carry out those commands, things will end badly for you. If you already have some doubts about that voice, the therapist may ask you not to complete the assignments for a week and carefully write down whether there are any negative consequences of your disobedience. If you attribute less power to votes, you will also be less bothered by them.

Examples of thoughts you may have about voices that are more bothering you:

The voices I hear are being produced by someone or something else.
The voices have power over me and I must obey them.
I can get rid of my voices by getting angry and yelling.
My voices can predict the future.
My voices know more than I do.
My voices have a personal meaning and purpose for me

Examples of thoughts you may have about voices that will make you less bothered:

The voices I hear are created in my head by a slightly disrupted process.
The voices are threatening, but they have no power over me. I don't have to obey them.
My voices diminish if I am not interested, scared or angry about it.
My voices only predict the future afterwards.
My voices only know what I know myself.
My voices are ultimately irrelevant.

Some patients are angry about what the voices are saying and desperately try to get rid of them by yelling or swearing. Angry, anxious sustained attention on the voices often makes them louder. Everything you pay attention to grows! Often patients overestimate the negative consequences and place great value on what the voices say. They have the idea: if the voices say bad things, then I must be no good. People can also fear loss of control: if the voices tell me something, then I can't resist. What can help is to accept the voices, just let them speak without overemphasizing them. Then you will notice that they become less intense. Anything you give little attention shrinks!

Meta-analyzes show that the effect size of cognitive behavioral therapy is small to medium and that the effects with voices are more pronounced than those with delusions. Compared to supportive conversations, cognitive behavioral therapy has a greater effect on positive symptoms (the effect size is approximately 0.23) and a significantly greater effect than only friendly conversations on total symptoms (the effect size is approximately 0.42) (Van der Gaag M et al., 2018).

How can you explain the development of a delusion?

In the cognitive explanatory model of psychosis, the formation of delusions is crucial. Hearing voices doesn't have to be a big deal in itself. Only because of the delusions about the origin, power and purpose of the voices does hearing them become problematic.

There are tendencies in how people process information that can encourage the development of delusions. One such tendency is "jumping to conclusions". Here you come to conclusions on the basis of very little information, and then you are strongly convinced of their correctness. In addition, many people tend to see causal relationships when in reality there is a coincidence. This tendency can also encourage the development of delusions. The human tendency to look for confirmatory information and to ignore contradictory information (so-called tunnel vision) also promotes the development of delusions. Tunnel vision is also common in people who do not have psychosis. Certain views about your own thinking can also cause problems. For example, if you think worrying can help you solve problems. Or if you think thoughts can be dangerous and uncontrollable on their own.

Certain perceptions of danger can also get you into trouble. You may see other people as a threat. Then you feel uncomfortable with others and tend to avoid them. Then you can develop a social phobia, where you fear that others will reject you, or you can become suspicious, where you fear that the other person will harm you. The fear makes you look for confirmation of what you already thought and you have the tendency to avoid "dangerous" situations, so that you never experience that it is not so bad.

When the above tendencies occur under stress and when more dopamine is released for a longer period, you become more and more convinced that special things are happening. Chapter 19 describes the role dopamine plays in this. In combination with those cognitive tendencies, you can then come to a catastrophic conclusion, such as that people are after you. From that moment on you avoid other people and you can even start barricading your door. In addition, your fear reinforces your selective attention to danger. Then you will avoid many situations in your life. You then constantly get anxious and sad memories and a negative self-image, while self-confidence and a positive self-image gets further away. You isolate yourself and no longer discuss your experiences and thoughts with others. As a result, others can no longer help you in mitigating your fears (Van der Gaag M et al., 2018).

What is Acceptance and Commitment Therapy [or ACT]?

ACT uses acceptance and mindfulness strategies, together with commitment and behavior change strategies, to increase psychological flexibility. ACT has a very simple effective philosophy. It is based on the idea that when you focus your attention on something it grows. Several core processes are important in ACT. Here I will describe a few. *Acceptance* is an alternative to our basic tendency to avoid thinking about negative- or potentially negative-experiences. It is the active choice to allow unpleasant experiences to exist, without trying to deny, control or change them. When you are able to accept negative thoughts or feelings, you no longer struggle with them and they will get less attention and shrink. *Cognitive Defusion* refers to the techniques intended to change how an individual reacts to their thoughts and feelings. You are not your thoughts. You have them. They can go away. They are not you. Acceptance and Commitment Therapy does not intend to limit your exposure to negative experiences or thoughts, but rather to face them without being attached to them. *Being Present* can be understood as the practice of being aware of the present moment, pay attention, without judging the experience. In other words, it involves experiencing what is happening without trying to change the experience.

Values are the qualities we choose to work towards in any given moment. We all hold values, consciously or unconsciously, that direct our steps. You are encouraged to focus on the things that you find really important in your life. Put the most of your effort and *commitment* on the things that are really valuable for you. ACT can help you to live your live in accordance with the values that you hold dear.

ACT is not very different from other behavioral-based therapies; it just emphasizes acceptance instead of avoidance, and in that way, is special.

ACT does not target specific symptoms in certain conditions, but negative thoughts and feelings that can affect anyone. Research shows that ACT helps with various problems. A small meta-analysis shows that there is no effect on the severity of symptoms in psychotic patients. New studies will appear in the foreseeable future. Recently, we found that ACT helps to improve social functioning and reduce the severity of negative symptoms. The idea behind this form of therapy is very clear. It's also a nice mix of

Eastern and Western wisdom. Try to accept what happens to you and commit to what you find valuable. I think this is one of the best therapeutic ideas available (Myin-Germeys I, et al. 2022).

Why can change be difficult?

We humans are creatures of habit. Once we are used to something or certain behavior, we tend to keep it that way. Change does not happen automatically. How did that happen? First, change requires willpower. You can also be afraid that the situation will not get better if you change. You might lose something that you were attached to. Maybe the new situation is not good for you at all. You can also be convinced that you are unable to change, or that you will quickly return to your old pattern. Many people who may want to change something are ambivalent: they think that change has advantages, but they also see disadvantages. That's why they stick with the old.

Yet change can also be good for you. Quitting cannabis use can help clear you up, reduce suspicion, improve your mood and help you concentrate. But on the other hand, you are afraid of losing friends or you don't know what to do without smoking. Starting to run can give you a boost. You get stronger, you feel fitter, your head becomes clearer and your mood improves. But how to get started! And how to persist? Not that simple. Motivational interviewing (see below) can help with this.

How come people have doubts about change?

People have doubts about change, because change creates tension between things that people consider important. On the one hand, people think about objections to change and about the effort that has been made. But on the other hand, also about what change can bring them and how well they would go. This doubt about what to decide is very common. You think it over again and again. Of course, you don't do that for nothing. You have doubts because change is about important things that can clash with each other. It's about things that you really value. On the one hand you want to be healthy, for example, but on the other hand you also want to have fun and enjoy yourself. That's called ambivalence. Often the result of this is that you do not start to change. You keep doubting and ambivalent, and everything stays the same. That is a condition suitable for motivational interviewing. By examining the advantages and disadvantages of a change in a conversation, you can gain clarity, you can think about what is most important to you.

What is motivational interviewing?

Motivational interviewing is a therapeutic technique that helps patients find motivation for change and gain confidence in their power to change. Motivational interviewing was created by William Miller and Stephen Rollnick. They were looking for a collaborative conversation style that strengthens someone's own motivation and willingness to change. The technique is therefore aimed at your own personal, inner motivation. In motivational interviews you explore the pros and cons of change together with your therapist, and together you try to find a solution for the ambivalence you feel. It is important that you yourself discover and name the arguments that may be of decisive importance. Only if you change your own thoughts, you have enough conviction. It doesn't help at all if you feel forced by a counselor or if someone else is trying to convince you. The point is that the friendly, safe and accepting attitude of the care provider allows you to think carefully about what you really want. This atmosphere of acceptance is very important in motivational conversations. It also makes sense that it must come from within yourself. You are the captain of your ship. You are the one who want to change (or not).

What are important elements of motivational interviewing?

Motivational interviewing has four core elements:

1. The care provider and the patient work together on the basis of equality. The patient is an expert in herself and her daily life. The counselor is an expert in her field.
2. The clinician accepts the patient's views and actions. The patient has autonomy and is ultimately the one who decides.
3. The care provider tries to promote the interests and well-being of the patient as well as possible. This is sometimes difficult. Care providers often have a preference for a certain change, because they think that this will best serve the patient's well-being (for example, that the patient stops smoking or that she continues to use antipsychotics). Compassion and acceptance can sometimes get in each other's way.
4. The care provider tries to purposefully investigate and understand the patient's thoughts and feelings, in order to discover and strengthen her inner motivation together with the patient.

How does a motivational interview generally proceed?

For a motivational interview, first and foremost, mutual trust must develop between the care provider and the patient. The rest will not work without trust. Second, there must be purpose in the conversation. It is not about small talk, you focus together. Then you will look for inner motivation together in the conversation. What do you want exactly? How can you put that into words? The counselor listens, asks questions and examines the pros and cons of change together with you. The care provider is of course not completely neutral. While he respects your autonomy, he encourages aspects that could lead to beneficial change. But the principle remains that it ultimately comes down to your inner consideration. Finally, the conversation focuses on making plans. How will you handle change? What is involved? How do you deal with possible barriers? What do you do if it doesn't work?

For what kinds of problems is motivational interviewing effective?

Positive effects of motivational interviewing have been found in different addictions (alcohol, cannabis, smoking) and in considering different treatment options.

Is motivational interviewing also effective in patients with a psychotic disorder?

There are indications that motivational interviewing is also effective in patients with a psychotic disorder. The choices for which motivational interviewing has been studied are the use of antipsychotics, drug use and healthy behavior. I will discuss some of the studies on these subjects below.

Does motivational interviewing help promote regular use of antipsychotics in patients with schizophrenia who have been admitted repeatedly because they developed new psychosis after they stopped taking antipsychotics?

Because we know that regular use of antipsychotics is a major source of distress in people who have had multiple psychotic episodes, it is important to know whether motivational interviewing can promote adherence. This was investigated by Emile Barkhof and his colleagues. They randomized 114 patients to five to eight sessions of motivational interviewing or to five to eight sessions of health education (this was the control group). Beside that, both groups received the same treatment. After 12 months, it was found that 27 percent of the patients who had received motivational interviewing had to be re-admitted compared to 40 percent in the control group (this difference was not significant, which means that it cannot be ruled out with 95 percent certainty that the finding was coincidental, yet the chances of it being a correct finding are quite high: about 81 percent). The effect was greater in women (9 percent versus 63 percent), as well as in patients who did not use cannabis (20 percent versus 53 percent) or were younger (14 percent versus 50 percent). In short, there are preliminary indications that motivational interviewing has beneficial effects in this group of chronic patients, especially in women, young people and people who do not use cannabis.

Is motivational interviewing effective in promoting antipsychotic depot treatment?

To investigate whether motivational interviewing can promote depot treatment with antipsychotics, 101 participants were randomized to regular treatment with psychoeducation and motivational interviewing and 101 participants to regular treatment. Fourteen patients from the group with psychoeducation and motivational interviewing and seven patients from the control group started using depot antipsychotics. Over the next year and a half, 13.9 percent of the participants in the psychoeducation and motivational interviewing group were re-admitted, while 22.8 percent of the control group participants were re-admitted. Psychoeducation and motivational interviewing therefore has a limited beneficial effect on re-admission.

In another study, 114 patients with schizophrenia spectrum disorders were randomized to eight sessions of motivational interviewing aimed at adherence to antipsychotics and regular care or to regular care only. After six months, patients from the group that had had motivational interviews appeared to use antipsychotics more often, to have a better understanding of the illness, to show fewer symptoms and to be hospitalized less often.

Does motivational interviewing ensure that patients with psychosis are more often present during cognitive training?

To find out whether motivational interviewing can increase the attendance of patients with psychosis in cognitive training, 64 patients were randomized to two sessions of motivational interviewing or two sessions of personal learning style (this was the control condition). Then it was assessed how often participants attended ten sessions of cognitive training. Motivational interviewing resulted in greater motivation and more training attendance.

Does short-term motivational interviewing help reduce drug use in patients with recent psychosis?

A small study found that thirteen patients who received motivational interviewing all reduced their drug use, while this happened in seven of the twelve patients in the control condition. The disadvantage of this study is that it is very small and that it was not randomized. The patients participating in the motivational interview were also more likely to live with family members, and this in itself may have reduced drug use.

Does it help parents to be trained in motivational interviewing to reduce cannabis use in young patients with schizophrenia?

Whether it helps to train parents in motivational conversations to reduce cannabis use in young patients with schizophrenia is a somewhat strange question at first glance: patients with schizophrenia use cannabis and you try to reduce that by training parents. But there is logic to this train of thought. If young people who have become psychotic continue to use cannabis, it often creates a lot of difficulties in contact with parents. Parents are angry and concerned, they want cannabis use to stop, and arguments often arise over cannabis use. But it often doesn't get any better, conflicts are substantial. Children smoking, Parents angry that smoking is being done. That is why Maarten Smeerdijk and others had the idea of teaching parents to deal with this problem differently, with the aim of reducing cannabis use in their children. This was investigated in a study in which 97 parents of 75 patients were randomized to training in motivational interviewing or to psychoeducation. Immediately after treatment and after fifteen months, children of parents who had learned motivational interviewing were clearly found to smoke less and less often. In other words, you don't have to be a professional to successfully practice motivational interviewing (Smeerdijk M, et al. 2012, 2015).

Is motivational interviewing effective in promoting healthy behavior in patients on long-term psychiatric treatment?

An uncontrolled study found that lifestyle intervention and motivational interviewing resulted in lower blood fat, fewer smokers and a decrease in symptom severity. That is a good result, but in this study there was no control group and there was (therefore) no randomization.

What is Mindfulness Training?

Mindfulness is a state of mind in which you are aware of your physical experiences, feelings and thoughts, without trying to change or control them. To achieve this state, you can practice meditation and other mindfulness exercises. Mindfulness is not a way to never experience stress or anxiety again, but it does help to deal with such inevitable feelings differently. Mindfulness training was originally Buddhist and then adapted in the United States to a therapy for stress reduction. The purpose of the training is to teach people to look at their experiences with mild, open attention.

A meta-analysis of the application of mindfulness training to different types of problems shows that if participants did mindfulness exercises for an average of eight weeks for about half an hour a day, they experienced less anxiety, depression and pain (effect size = 0.38), and that their quality of life improves slightly (effect size = 0.30). After a few months, this favorable effect diminished.

There is no agreement on the effects of mindfulness training in psychosis. Chinese research has shown mindfulness to be quite effective, but four European studies do not show a clear favorable result. This could be because the standard treatment in Europe is better than in China. With good standard treatment, it is more difficult for a new therapy to do it even better.

What is Competitive Memory Training?

Even if you know that voices have no power, you can still think about bad things every time you hear them. When the voices say you're a fool, you can think of all the times you were stupid or thought stupid in the past. The content of the voices is then directly related to sad or fearful memories. Competitive Memory Training (COMET) tries to associate the voices with the exact opposite of these bad memories. The intention is to make the connection with anxious and depressive memories less strong. First, the predominant theme of the votes is mapped. When that negative theme is clear, a strong example of a positive counterpart is sought.

Suppose the negative theme is that you are a loser. Then, as counterparts, memories are recalled of moments of success. You got your driver's license. Scored a goal. You made a good joke. These memories are discussed in detail and you try to relive them. As a result, you impress them strongly in your memory. This allows you to quickly retrieve these memories. When you bring back that pleasant emotion and at the same time imagine that you are hearing the voices, you will practice holding on to your enjoyable emotion.

Randomized controlled research has shown that with this therapy the voices do not decrease, but are perceived as less powerful, and that voices are seen less as caused by others outside yourself. This increases self-esteem (Van der Gaag M et al., 2018).

What are new developments in cognitive behavioral therapy?

Thinking about psychotherapy is influenced by a new theory about the development and persistence of psychological complaints: network theory. Here, the idea is that one symptom can increase the likelihood of another symptom developing, causing another symptom to develop, and so on.

Imagine worrying because you think you made the wrong decision. That worrying makes you fall asleep late. You wake up tired, have less energy, you do your job less well and you are short with friends. Your friends react less pleasantly to you and your colleagues are less satisfied with you, your mood continues to drop, which makes you worry even more, sleep worse and eventually depression develops. Network theory assumes that one symptom provokes another. But that also provides insight into psychotherapeutic possibilities. If you could reduce an important symptom, the stimulating effect on other symptoms would disappear and the "clinical picture" could clear up. Network theory also explains why so many problems do not adhere to characteristics of the DSM-5. Worrying occurs in anxiety disorders, depression, psychosis, and just in everyone's life.

In recent years, a number of short-term cognitive-behavioral therapy interventions targeting one specific factor have proven effective. It is often found that the effective treatment of one factor in the "psychopathology network" ensures that other complaints also improve. Some examples:

In seven sessions, patients with psychosis retrieved positive qualities from themselves with lively examples. This improved self-image, reduced psychosis symptoms and also improved social functioning.

A meta-analysis showed that a short intervention is effective in reducing insomnia. This also reduced suspicion.

Short-term anti-worry interventions have also been shown to be effective in reducing both worry and suspicion in the long term.

What is Cognitive Behavioral Therapy with Virtual Reality?

Behavioral experiments and exercises can be done in real life, but nowadays also in an interactive virtual world with virtual reality glasses on. Although these virtual worlds do not exactly resemble reality, they evoke similar emotional responses and can also cause, for instance, paranoid thoughts. Advantages of practicing in a virtual world is that the practice situation can be tailor-made and that you can practice in the treatment room while the therapist supports you. Virtual Cognitive Behavioral Therapy is modestly effective in reducing anxiety and paranoid thoughts (effect sizes 0.29 and 0.33, respectively).

What is Cognitive Rehabilitation?

Cognitive rehabilitation is a training program aimed at the rehabilitation of cognitive functions. There are two forms of training. In the first place, fitness training, in which a cognitive function is trained through a lot of repetition. For example, you can train your speed of reaction behind the computer. After a few weeks of training, the speed of reaction of participants has increased. But it is uncertain whether this also helps in daily functioning. In the second place, strategy training, where you learn a new strategy to deal with something that bothers you. Suppose you do not easily perceive directly that someone is anxious. Then you can learn to recognize this emotion in others when you know that fear is the only emotion where the white of the eye is visible above the iris. Some meta-analyzes do find a beneficial effect of cognitive rehabilitation, others do not. It depends which studies are included. So, there is little consistent evidence.

References

Myin-Germeys I, et al. Efficacy of Acceptance and Commitment Therapy in Daily Life in Early Psychosis: Results from the Multi-Center INTERACT Randomized Controlled Trial. Psychother Psychosom. 2022;91(6):411-423.

Smeerdijk M, et al. Motivational interviewing and interaction skills training for parents to change cannabis use in young adults with recent-onset schizophrenia: a randomized controlled trial. Psychol Med. 2012 Aug;42(8):1627-36.

Smeerdijk M, et al. Motivational interviewing and interaction skills training for parents of young adults with recent-onset schizophrenia and co-occurring cannabis use: 15-month follow-up. Psychol Med. 2015 Oct;45(13):2839-48.

Van der Gaag M et al., 2018. "Psychotherapie" In Handboek schizofreniespectrumstoornissen, edited by Wiepke Cahn, Inez Myin-Germeys, Richard Bruggeman, Lieuwe de Haan. Amsterdam: De Tijdstroom.

CHAPTER 43

PHYSICAL ACTIVITY

Why is physical activity important?

Physical activities can be a lot of fun, feel good and boost your self-confidence. Being physically active is good for your physical and mental health. People with schizophrenia are more likely to have physical and mental problems, so physical activity has additional benefits for them. Regarding the physical benefits, it helps you feel better, your physical health improves and it reduces the risk of cardiovascular disease. In general, people with schizophrenia have a two to three times higher risk of dying from cardiovascular disease. The risk of cardiovascular disease is increased by smoking, weight gain (common with antipsychotics) and unhealthy diet, and lack of physical activity. Physical activity is also good for your mental health. Meta-analyzes have shown that it greatly improves positive, negative and especially depressive symptoms. Moreover, it has a beneficial effect on cognitive functioning and your quality of life. Exercise is good for you!

Do people with schizophrenia exercise too little?

Just over half of people with schizophrenia meet the health recommendation of 150 minutes of physical activity every week of at least moderate intensity. That means that slightly less than half moves too little. Now the "normal" population on average also moves too little. However, a meta-analysis shows that people with schizophrenia are less physically active than the general population. They move less with moderate intensity (effect size about -0.45) and they move less with high intensity (effect size about -0.39). Moreover, patients with psychosis sit more than eleven hours a day on average, which is almost three hours more than the average population.

Why do people with schizophrenia exercise so little?

The fact that people with schizophrenia exercise so little can be due to many different factors: pain and physical discomfort, sleeping problems, lack of energy, special body experiences, negative symptoms, depressive symptoms, a lack of knowledge about the risks of little exercise, lack of knowledge of the benefits of physical activity, fear of the outside world, no reason to go outside, low self-confidence and lack of social support. Some of these causes can be addressed. Some factors are made worse by too little exercise. For example, your condition decreases if you are not physically active and as a result you have less energy. That is a nasty vicious circle.

What evidence is there for the beneficial effect of physical activity on the physical health of people with schizophrenia?

Meta-analyzes of research in people with schizophrenia show that physical activity improves heart and lung fitness (effect size approximately 0.43). The mean increase in maximal oxygen capacity, the best measure of heart and lung fitness, is 2.87 ml / kg / min. Such an improvement reduces the risk of premature death from cardiovascular disease by about 15 percent. It was striking that the meta-analysis showed no significant decrease in body mass index (BMI; the weight divided by the square of your height) (mean difference = -1.0 kg / m2). Yet even with the same weight, there is a beneficial effect. The amount of belly fat decreases through physical activity, and the amount of belly fat in particular is associated with the risk of cardiovascular disease. Your muscles become stronger and your muscle mass increases (moreover, muscles are heavier than fat). As a result, your weight does not decrease that much when you move more. But you look more healthy (Vancampfort D et al 2018).

What evidence is there for the beneficial effect of physical activity on the mental health of people with schizophrenia?

Meta-analyzes have shown that physical activity improves positive, negative and depressive symptoms (mean effect size on all these symptoms is approximately 0.40). In cognitive functioning, improvements were found in working memory (effect size = 0.39), attention (effect size = 0.66) and social cognition (effect size = 0.71). No significant effect was found in the other cognitive domains. General functioning and quality of life did improve. The magnitude of these effects is considerable: equal to or greater than the most effective forms of psychotherapy or medication! It is therefore advisable not to miss this opportunity for improvement (Vancampfort D et al 2018).

How intensively do you have to exercise to get these great benefits?

To get these great benefits, you need to be physically active at least three times a week for half an hour at moderate intensity. A moderate intensity is accompanied by an increase in heart rate and breathing due to the effort (you should no longer be able to talk to each other very easily). You achieve this by running, swimming or cycling briskly for half an hour three times a week, or by working with weights. But of course, you can play football, skating or basketball just as well. Mind you, also less intensive forms of exercise are beneficial. Cycling or walking more slowly also has beneficial effects on your well-being and your mental and physical health, although the effects may be a little less.

What is the problem with physical activity in people with schizophrenia?

Changing behavior is difficult for everyone. You have to cross a threshold and you have to continue. That can be tricky. That it can be difficult to motivate people with schizophrenia to maintain physical activity is also shown by a meta-analysis, according to which about 25 percent of participants stopped physical activity before the end of the analyzed studies. On the other hand, it is of course the case that 75 percent did survive.

What can be done to avoid giving up physical activity?

One study showed that counseling by physiotherapists, psychomotor therapists, sports scientists or sports doctors helped to prevent nearly two-thirds of the dropout. This is probably because these professionals take physical and psychiatric complaints into account when making a so-called exercise plan.

It also helps enormously to exercise with someone else or in a group.

It is important to take into account everyone's need for autonomy, competence and social belonging in the physical activity plan:

Regarding autonomy: you want to keep the feeling that you decide and determine what you do. That is why freedom of choice in the exercise plan is very important. You have to do something that suits you.

Regarding competence: you want to feel that you are achieving what you want and you feel able to do so. Usually, people manage to achieve goals that they think in advance have a 70 percent chance of success. You can take this into account when setting your goals.

Regarding social connection: you want to be involved with others in a meaningful way. Exercising together in a group in which you feel accepted is very rewarding.

What also appears to help: discuss with a therapist the benefits and obstacles of exercise and find out how you can tackle those obstacles in real life (Vancampfort D et al 2018).

When should it be checked whether exercise is medically justified?

Sometimes you have to be careful with physical exercise. If you have pain or a heart or lung disease, or if you have pain during exercise or have had severe shortness of breath or palpitations, for example. If you answer "yes" to any of the following seven questions, it is wise to consult a doctor before you start exercising:

1. Has a doctor ever said that you have a heart problem?
2. Do you have chest pain during physical exertion?
3. In the past month, have you had chest pain when you were not doing any physical activity?
4. Do you ever lose your balance due to dizziness or do you ever lose consciousness?
5. Do you have a skeletal or joint problem (for example, of the back, knee or hip) that can be made worse by physical activity?
6. Is your doctor currently prescribing medication for your blood pressure or a heart problem?
7. Are you aware of any other reasons why you should be careful about physical exercise?

References

Vancampfort D et al 2018. "Fysieke activiteit" In Handboek schizofreniespectrumstoornissen, edited by Wiepke Cahn, Inez Myin-Germeys, Richard Bruggeman, Lieuwe de Haan. Amsterdam: De Tijdstroom.

CHAPTER 44

NEUROSTIMULATION

What is Neurostimulation?

Neurostimulation is a form of treatment in which neural processing is influenced via electric current or a magnetic field.

What forms of neurostimulation have been studied in controlled studies in schizophrenia?

Electroconvulsive therapy (ECT) and transcranial magnetic stimulation (TMS) are two forms of neurostimulation that have been studied in schizophrenia. The effect of neurostimulation is temporary. Maintenance treatment is necessary to maintain the effect.

What forms of neurostimulation still need to be investigated before they can possibly be used in schizophrenia?

Transcranial Direct Current Stimulation (TDCS) or DC modulation has been shown to be effective in depression, with hardly any side effects (transient mild headache or itching). Some uncontrolled studies also show favorable results for psychotic symptoms, negative symptoms and catatonia. TDCS in itself can be examined double-blind, because the treatment is not immediately noticeable. In addition, TDCS is a simple technique that could even be applied by a patient himself. We are awaiting more investigation (Koop S and Sommer I 2018).

What is Transcranial Magnetic Stimulation?

In transcranial magnetic stimulation, a magnetic field influences local brain activity. By passing electrical current through a coil of copper wire and holding it above the patient's head, a magnetic field with a strength of 1 to 3 Tesla is created. This affects the activity of neurons in a small area of the brain (about the size of a table tennis ball). The activity of this brain area can therefore be temporarily inhibited or, on the contrary, stimulated (Koop S and Sommer I 2018).

What problems is TMS used for?

In the United States, TMS is approved for the treatment of depression, and some health insurers in the Netherlands reimburse the TMS treatment for hearing voices. A repeating TMS pulse per second is given for about twenty minutes. Recent meta-analyzes show an effect size of 0.29 to 0.44 on the severity of hallucinations. TMS may affect negative and cognitive symptoms, but further research is needed (Koop S and Sommer I 2018).

What else needs to be investigated regarding TMS?

Further research is needed into why some patients benefit greatly from TMS treatment, while others experience no effect at all. There may be large differences in individual sensitivity to the strength of the TMS signal.

When is electroconvulsive therapy suitable?

If someone continues to experience significant problems with positive symptoms despite adequate treatment with clozapine, ECT is suitable. A recent meta-analysis with 1769 patients in a randomized controlled trial showed that the combination of clozapine and ECT works better than treatment with clozapine alone. The effect size is 0.54. There is methodological criticism concerning the studies included in this meta-analysis. For example, the studies are not placebo controlled. It is also difficult to keep patients blind to the ECT. The methodological quality of these studies could be improved when the person who measures the severity of the symptoms does not know who has and who has not received ECT. With the current research we can state that ECT has added value, but that we cannot entirely rule out the possibility that this added value is partly based on a placebo effect (Koop S and Sommer I 2018).

How is ECT applied?

With ECT, a patient is briefly anesthetized and a muscle relaxant is administered. Then an epileptic seizure (so-called convulsion) is induced by means of an electric current. ECT often has to be applied several days a week for several weeks in a row before the effect is noticeable.

Figure 44.1 ECT

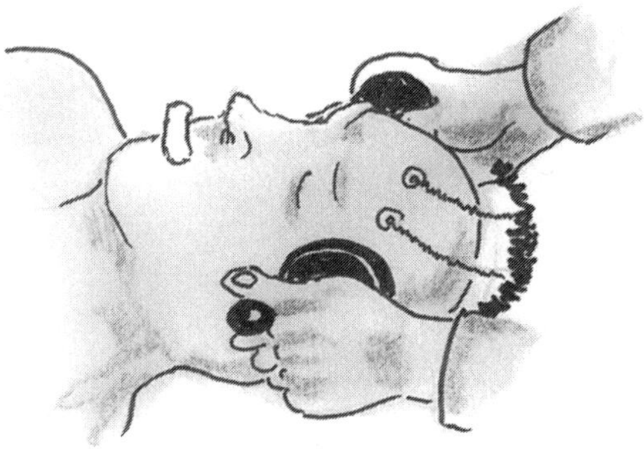

What are side effects of ECT?

Side effects of ECT include headaches, temporary confusion, temporary amnesia, and difficulty storing new information. ECT also causes a short absence of cardiac activity. During the epileptic seizure there is an increased activity of the autonomic nervous system. The aforementioned metanalysis showed that ECT is usually well tolerated and that the headaches and memory problems were not serious and almost always passed. A recent review article described that a number of studies even found improvement of cognitive functioning during ECT (Koop S and Sommer I 2018).

References

Koop S and Sommer I 2018. "Neurostimulatie" In Handboek schizofreniespectrumstoornissen, edited by Wiepke Cahn, Inez Myin-Germeys, Richard Bruggeman, Lieuwe de Haan. Amsterdam: De Tijdstroom.